Enteral Nutrition

CHAPMAN & HALL SERIES IN CLINICAL NUTRITION

Ronni Chernoff, Ph.D., R.D.
Series Editor

Enteral Nutrition
Bradley C. Borlase, M.D., M.S.
Stacey J. Bell, M.S., R.D., CNSD
George L. Blackburn, M.D., Ph.D.
R. Armour Forse, M.D., Ph.D.

Pediatric Enteral Nutrition
Susan S. Baker, M.D., Ph.D.
Robert Baker, M.D., Ph.D.
Anne Davis, M.S., R.D., CNSD

Obesity: Pathophysiology, Psychology, and Treatment
George L. Blackburn, M.D., Ph.D.
Beatrice S. Kanders, Ed.D., M.P.H., R.D.

ENTERAL NUTRITION

Chapman & Hall Series in Clinical Nutrition
Series Editor: Ronni Chernoff, Ph.D., R.D.

Edited by

Bradley C. Borlase, M.D., M.S.
Harvard Medical School, New England Deaconess Hospital

Stacey J. Bell, M.S., R.D., C.N.S.D.
New England Deaconess Hospital

George L. Blackburn, M.D., Ph.D.
Harvard Medical School, New England Deaconess Hospital

R. Armour Forse, M.D., Ph.D.
Harvard Medical School, New England Deaconess Hospital

CHAPMAN
& HALL

No responsibility is assumed by the Publisher for any injury and/or damage to persons or property as a matter of products liability, negligence or otherwise, or from any use or operation of any methods, products, instructions or ideas contained in the material herein. No suggested test or procedure should be carried out unless, in the reader's judgment, its risk is justified. Because of rapid advances in the medical sciences, we recommend that independent verification of diagnoses and drug dosages should be made. Discussion, views, and recommendations as to medical procedures, choice of drugs, and drug dosages are the responsibility of the authors.

First published in 1994 by
Chapman & Hall
One Penn Plaza
New York, NY 10119

Published in Great Britain by
Chapman & Hall
2–6 Boundary Row
London SE1 8HN

Printed in the United States of America

©1994 Chapman & Hall, Inc.

All rights reserved. No part of this book may be reprinted or reproduced or utilized in any form or by any electronic, mechanical or other means, now known or hereafter invented, including photocopying and recording, or by an information storage or retrieval system, without permission in writing from the publishers.

Library of Congress Cataloging-in-Publication Data

Enteral nutrition / Bradley C. Borlase ... [et al].
    p. cm—(Chapman & Hall series in clinical nutrition)
  Includes bibliographical references.
  ISBN 0-412-98471-7
  1. Enteral feeding. I. Borlase, Bradley C. II. Series.
RM225.E578 1994
615.8'55–dc20
    93-47999
    CIP

British Library Cataloguing in Publication Data available

Please send your order for this or any other Chapman & Hall book to **Chapman & Hall, 29 West 35th Street, New York, NY 10001, Attn: Customer Service Department.** You may also call our Order Department at 1-212-244-3336 or fax your purchase order to 1-800-248-4724.

For a complete listing of Chapman & Hall's titles, send your request to **Chapman & Hall, Dept. BC, One Penn Plaza, New York, NY 10119.**

Contents

Foreword ix

Preface xi

Contributors xiii

PART I SCIENTIFIC RATIONALE FOR ENTERAL NUTRITION

Chapter 1 Gastrointestinal Physiology and the Gastrointestinal Tract as a Central Organ in the Hypermetabolic Response to Injury 3
Kirth W. Steele, D.O., Douglas L. Seidner, M.D., and *Gordon L. Jensen, M.D., Ph.D.*

Chapter 2	Bacterial Translocation *Jason G. Nirgiotis, M.D.* and *Richard J. Andrassy, M.D., F.A.C.S.*	15
Chapter 3	Enteral Nutrition and Critical Illness *John L. Rombeau, M.D.*	25
Chapter 4	Requirements for Patients Receiving Enteral Nutrition *Scott Shikora, M.D.*	37
Chapter 5	Specific Nutrients for the Gastrointestinal Tract: Glutamine, Arginine, Nucleotides, and Structured Lipids *Timothy J. Babineau, M.D.*	47
PART II	CLINICAL RATIONALE AND TECHNIQUES FOR ENTERAL NUTRITION	
Chapter 6	A Successful Technique for Providing Enteral Nutrition *Bradley C. Borlase, M.D., M.S., Stacey J. Bell, M.S., R.D., CNSD, R. Armour Forse, M.D., Ph.D.,* and *George L. Blackburn, M.D., Ph.D.*	63
Chapter 7	Development of an Enteral Nutrition Support Service *Stacey J. Bell, M.S., R.D., CNSD, Bradley C. Borlase, M.D., M.S., Wendy Swails, R.D., Kathy Dascoulias, D.T.R.,* and *R. Armour Forse, M.D., Ph.D.*	69
Chapter 8	Early Postoperative Feeding *Todd N. Jones, M.S., R.N., CNSN, Ernest E. Moore, M.D.,* and *Frederick A. Moore, M.D.*	78
Chapter 9	Transitional Feeding *Elaine Barbella Trujillo, M.S., R.D., CNSD,* and *Patricia M. Queen, R.D.*	107

Chapter 10	Selecting Enteral Products *Patrick Pasulka, M.D., F.A.C.P.,* and *Christine Crockett, R.D., CNSD*	115
Chapter 11	Early Enteral Feeding via a Feeding Jejunostomy: A Safe Technique in Critically Ill Patients *Thomas L. Khoury, M.D., Bradley C. Borlase, M.D., M.S., R. Armour Forse, M.D., Ph.D., Stacey J. Bell, M.S., R.D., CNSD, Wendy Swails, R.D., CNSD., George L. Blackburn, M.D., Ph.D.,* and *Bruce R. Bistrian, M.D., Ph.D.*	142

PART III PRACTICAL APPLICATIONS FOR ENTERAL NUTRITION

Chapter 12	Who Should Receive Enteral Nutrition and What Are the Nutrient Requirements? *Martha Lebow, R.D.*	155
Chapter 13	Micronutrient Additives *Wendy Swails, R.D., CNSD*	161
Chapter 14	Enteral Feeding Formulas and Administrative Techniques *Patricia Heanue, R.D.*	173
Chapter 15	Metabolic Complications *Kelli Guenther, R.D., CNSD*	181
Chapter 16	Gastrointestinal Complications: Diarrhea and High Gastric Residuals *Shanthi Thomas, M.S., R.D., CNSD*	188
Chapter 17	Feeding Tube Placement *Bradley C. Borlase, M.D., M.S.,* and *R. Armour Forse, M.D., Ph.D.*	193
Chapter 18	Care of Feeding Tubes *Ann Thibault, R.N., CNSN*	197

Chapter 19	Transitional Feeding Strategies for Discharge *Elaine B. Trujillo, M.S., R.D., CNSD*	199
	Index	207

Foreword

Advances in clinical nutrition seem to be occurring with increasing frequency as we approach the end of the twentieth century. With the imminent overhaul of the country's health care system, practitioners who are committed to providing the highest quality care should pay close attention to the value of nutrition. With these factors in mind, Chapman & Hall launched a series of books that address special topics in clinical nutrition. Through this series we hope to provide texts that explore, in depth, specific topics in nutrition that give the practitioner the scientific basis for the interventions described, and practical discussions of how to apply these interventions. Our hope is to provide quality texts that are timely, thorough, and well written by authors who are recognized experts in their fields.

Enteral Nutrition, edited by Bradley C. Borlase, Stacey J. Bell, George L. Blackburn, and R. Armour Forse, is the first in a series on clinical nutrition. This volume is divided into three parts. The first part discusses the scientific rationale for enteral nutrition. It addresses the gastrointestinal (GI) tract and its function as an organ, particularly its responses to injury and illness. To aid in the successful use of enteral feeding as an intervention, it describes the physiology and the functioning of the GI tract in great detail. It also reviews new information on specific nutrients that have unique roles in the GI tract.

The second part of the book addresses the clinical rationale and practical techniques for successfully delivering enteral nutrition. Along with useful information on techniques for early postoperative feeding, transitional feeding, and nursing considerations, it provides important information on developing and maintaining an enteral nutrition support service. This information is necessary to guarantee the most efficient, most effective, and highest quality care. These chapters were written specifically to give the healthcare professional an understanding of the rationale for many of the activities that are needed to manage enteral nutrition support successfully.

The third part of the book was designed as a handbook for performing the activities associated with delivering enteral nutrition. The chapters in this section describe the indications for enteral feeding, formulas and various additives, complications (metabolic and gastrointestinal), feeding tubes, and transitional feedings. This part of the book includes everything a novice practioner needs to know.

Often, those practitioners who are experienced in the art and science of enteral feeding forget that very few health care practitioners, regardless of discipline, are as accomplished as they are. There is a constant need to educate individuals new to the field. This need can be met through books that present comprehensive discussions of various topics. This book offers the scientific rationale for feeding patients by tube and, at the same time, describes what can be accomplished with a sound, practical approach to the delivery, monitoring, and management of enteral nutrition. It is a much needed reference for all healthcare practitioners (physicians, dietitians, nurses, and pharmacists) who engage in the art and science of dispensing nutrition intervention to patients in need.

Ronni Chernoff, Ph.D., R.D.
Series Editor, Chapman & Hall Series in Clinical Nutrition

Preface

The use of enteral nutrition support has increased both because of improvements in formulas and delivery systems and because clinicians now have a greater appreciation of its merits in preserving gastrointestinal function and minimizing infections related to enteric pathogens. Despite this growth of enthusiasm, however, several reports in the literature discuss complications associated with this route of feeding. Although many of these are not necessarily life threatening (e.g., diarrhea, gastrointestinal discomfort), they often preclude the patient from receiving a full day's nutrition. This book was developed by our Nutrition Support Service and others who appreciate the merits of enteral support.

This book details both the scientific rationale for using enteral feeding and the practical approach used by our group and others around the country. The first two parts review current topics of interest in the field: bacterial translocation (Andrassy), enteral feeding and critical illness (Rombeau), the gastrointestinal tract (Jensen), early postoperative feeding (Moore), and formula selection (Pasulka).

The last part, written by the Enteral Nutrition Service of our Nutritional Support Service, the Enteral Nutritional Service, covers topics that come up daily at rounds. Issues discussed include nutrient requirements, formula selection, administrative techniques, diarrhea management, and transition to home care. Each chapter answers one of the most frequently asked questions about the enteral feeding of hospitalized and home patients.

This book is for anyone who provides enteral nutrition to hospitalized or home patients, including physicians, dietitians, nurses, and pharmacists. The chapters were written by members of these disciplines to summarize the particular areas of interest within each field.

Bradley C. Borlase, M.D., M.S.
Stacey J. Bell, M.S., R.D., CNSD
George L. Blackburn, M.D., Ph.D.
R. Armour Forse, M.D., Ph.D.

Contributors

Richard J. Andrassy, M.D.
A.G. McNeese Professor of Pediatric Surgery
The Division of Pediatric Surgery
The University of Texas Medical School at Houston and the MD Anderson Cancer Center
6431 Fannin, Suite 6264
Houston, TX 77030

Timothy J. Babineau, M.D.
Instructor in Surgery
Harvard Medical School
Nutrition Support Service
Department of Surgery
New England Deaconess Hospital
110 Francis Street, Suite 3A
Boston, MA 02215

Stacey J. Bell, M.S., R.D., CNSD
Nutrition Support Service
New England Deaconess Hospital
194 Pilgrim Road
Boston, MA 02215

Bruce R. Bistrian, M.D., Ph.D.
Professor of Medicine
Harvard Medical School
Chief, Nutrition/Infection Laboratory
New England Deaconess Hospital
194 Pilgrim Road
Boston, MA 02215

George L. Blackburn, M.D., Ph.D.
Associate Professor of Surgery
Harvard Medical School
Chief, Nutrition/Metabolism
  Laboratory
New England Deaconess Hospital
194 Pilgrim Road
Boston, MA 02215

Bradley C. Borlase, M.D., M.S.
Former Instructor in Surgery
Harvard Medical School
New England Deaconess Hospital
110 Francis Street, Suite 3A
Boston, MA 02215

Christine Crockett, R.D., CNSD
Clinical Dietitian
Nutritional Support Service
Good Samaritan Regional Medical
  Center
Phoenix, AZ 85004

Kathleen J. Dascoulias, D.T.R.
Nutrition Support Service
New England Deaconess Hospital
194 Pilgrim Road
Boston, MA 02215

R. Armour Forse, M.D., Ph.D.
Assistant Professor of Surgery
Harvard Medical School
Chief, Surgical Metabolism
  Laboratory
Department of Surgery
New England Deaconess Hospital
194 Pilgrim Road
Boston, MA 02215

Kelli Guenther, R.D., CNSD
Staff Dietitian
New England Deaconess Hospital
194 Pilgrim Road
Boston, MA 02215

Patricia Heanue, R.D.
Staff Dietitian
New England Deaconess
  Hospital
194 Pilgrim Road
Boston, MA 02215

Gordon L. Jensen, M.D., Ph.D.
Associate Professor of Medicine
Departments of Critical Care
  Medicine and Gastroenterology
  and Nutrition
Geisner Medical Center
Danville, PA 17822

Todd N. Jones, M.S., R.N.,
  CNSN
Clinical Nutrition Specialist
McGraw, Inc.
2525 McGaw Avenue
P.O. Box 19791
Irvine, CA 92713-9791

Thomas L. Khoury, M.D.
Former Clinical Fellow in
  Hyperalimentation and
  Metabolism
Harvard Medical School
New England Deaconess
  Hospital
194 Pilgrim Road
Boston, MA 02215

Martha Lebow, R.D.
Staff Dietician
New England Deaconess Hospital
194 Pilgrim Road
Boston, MA 02215

Ernest E. Moore, M.D.
Chief, Department of Surgery
Denver General Hospital
777 Bannock Street
Denver, CO 80204

Fredrick A. Moore, M.D.
Chief, Critical Care
Denver General Hospital
777 Bannock Street
Denver, CO 80204

Jason G. Nirgiotis, M.D.
The Division of Pediatric Surgery
The University of Texas Medical School at Houston and the MD Anderson Cancer Center
6431 Fannin, Suite 6264
Houston, TX 77030

Patrick Pasulka, M.D., F.A.C.P.
Assistant Clinical Professor of Medicine
University of Arizona Medical Center
Director, Nutrition Support Service
Good Samaritan Regional Medical Center
Phoenix, AZ 85004

Patricia Queen, R.D.
Director, Department of Clinical Dietetics
New England Deaconess Hospital
194 Pilgrim Road
Boston, MA 02215

John L. Rombeau, M.D.
Associate Professor of Surgery
Department of Surgery
Hospital of the University of Pennsylvania
3400 Spruce Street
Philadelphia, PA 19104

Douglas L. Seidner, M.D.
Departments of Critical Care Medicine and Gastroenterology and Nutrition
Geisner Medical Center
Danville, PA 17822

Scott Shikora, M.D.
Department of Surgery
Wilford Hall—USAF Medical Center
Lackland AFB, TX 78236-5300

Kirth W. Steele, D.O.
Departments of Critical Care Medicine and Gastroenterology and Nutrition
Geisner Medical Center
Danville, PA 17822

Wendy Swails, R.D.
Research Dietitian
New England Deaconess Hospital
194 Pilgrim Road
Boston, MA 02215

Ann Thibault, R.N., CNSN
Nutrition Support Service
New England Deaconess Hospital
194 Pilgrim Road
Boston, BA 02215

Shanti Thomas, M.S., CNSD
Nutrition Support RD
Brockton Hospital
Brockton, MA 02302

Elaine Barbella Trujillo, M.S., R.D., CNSD
Nutrition Support RD
Brigham and Womens Hospital
Boston, MA 02115

PART I

SCIENTIFIC RATIONALE FOR ENTERAL NUTRITION

Gastrointestinal Physiology and the Gastrointestinal Tract as a Central Organ in the Hypermetabolic Response to Injury

CHAPTER 1

Kirth W. Steele, D.O., Douglas L. Seidner, M.D., and Gordon L. Jensen, M.D., Ph.D.

INTRODUCTION

The gastrointestinal tract was once believed to be a passive conduit for nutrient absorption that functioned suboptimally in the critically ill patient and could easily be bypassed through the use of parenteral nutrition. It is now evident that the gut plays a central role in the injury response and that the maintenance of normal gut function and integrity through enteral feeding and the provision of conditionally essential nutrients may hasten recovery and improve survival.

Normal digestion and absorption form a complex process by which food is broken down into simple amino acids, sugars, and fatty acids that gain entry into the portal vein or intestinal lymphatics. This process begins in the oral cavity where solids are masticated and starch digestion is initiated by salivary amylase. Peristaltic activity within the stomach increases food surface area, while acid and pepsin initiate breakdown of protein. The processing of triglycerides may begin with salivary and gastric lipases, but it is not until the proximal small bowel that pancreatic lipase, colipase, and bile salts complete triglyceride digestion. Mixed micelles of fatty acids, partial glycerides, and bile salts are then absorbed by the enterocyte. The majority of polypeptide and oligosaccharide digestion occurs as a result of pancreatic enzymes, with final breakdown occurring by brush-border peptidases and disaccharidases.

ENTEROCYTE FUNCTION AND INJURY

The enterocyte is highly susceptible to injury, so nutrient assimilation and other gut functions may be impaired in the critically ill patient. The incidence of gastrointestinal failure reportedly varies from 7 to 30% (1), but the pathogenesis of this process has been difficult to define and characterize and the true incidence of enterocyte dysfunction is probably underestimated. The turnover of enterocytes is a dynamic process that begins in the crypt region with an undifferentiated stem cell and proceeds until the mature cell reaches the tip of the intestinal villous (2). Many factors regulate this process.

The presence of food in the small bowel plays an integral role in the maintenance of normal villous architecture and function. Animals fed orally have higher gut weights, mucosal thickness, protein and DNA contents, disaccharidase activity, and epithelial cell proliferation than animals fed intravenously (3,4). When animals are subjected to massive small bowel resection, only those fed enterally exhibit appreciable mucosal growth and functional adaptation (5,6). In addition to the nutritive effects of food, there appears to be some degree of cellular proliferation, on the basis of mechanical stimulation by nonnutrient foodstuff (7) and dietary fiber (8).

Gastric, duodenal, and pancreaticobiliary secretions have been shown to stimulate cellular proliferation and increase villous height (9). This effect may result from the release of free amino acids by protein digestion (10), or alterations in mucosal permeability due to chronic irritation of intestinal epithelium (11). Cholecystokinin and secretin are released in response to dietary protein, fat, or decreased luminal pH, and may prevent hypoplasia through the release of pancreaticobiliary secretions (10).

Hormonal and neurovascular factors may play a role in stimulating or inhibiting epithelial cell growth. Loran et al. postulated the existence of an "intestinal epithelial growth hormone" (12). Hormones implicated include gastrin (13), glucagon (14), mineralocorticoids (15), pituitary hormones (16), testosterone (17), thyroxin (18), serotonin (18), histamine (18), and enteroglucagon (19). Stimulation of mesenteric nerves electrically or by cholinergic drugs has been shown to stimulate intestinal cell proliferation (18).

The enterocyte serves as the barrier between the sterile interstitial and intracellular environments and the body's bacteria-laden external environment. This barrier is made up of a single layer of cells that are in a constant state of turnover. The process of differentiation, maturation, and ultimate desquamation takes only

TABLE 1-1. Characteristics of Hypermetabolism

Hemodynamic	Hormonal	Protein	Carbohydrate	Fat
↑ CO	↑ Cortisol	↓ Total synthesis	↑ Gluconeogenesis	↑ Lipolysis
↓ SVR	↑ Glucagon	↑ Catabolism	↑ Lactate	↓ Lipogenesis
↓ A–$\overline{V}O_2$	↑ Insulin	↑ Liver synthesis		↓ Ketosis
	↑ Epinephrine	↑ Ureagenesis		
	↓ Growth hormone			
	↓ T_3, T_4			

CO, cardiac output; SVR, systemic vascular resistance; A–$\overline{V}O_2$, arterial/mixed venous oxygen content difference.

a few days. Because of this rapid cellular turnover, an enormous amount of energy is required in a constant, uninterrupted supply. Utilization of this energy requires oxygen and essential cellular nutrients. If the energy flow is interrupted (i.e., trauma, stress, injury), the stage is set for cell death, loss of barrier function, translocation of bacteria and endotoxin, and release of mediators leading to multiple organ failure and death. The syndrome of multiple organ failure probably represents a continuum along an axis illustrated by injury–response–hypermetabolism–organ failure–death.

After an injury or stress, there are a series of well-defined responses by the organism that were first described by Cuthbertson (20,21) over 50 years ago. Immediately following an injury, extracellular fluid sequestration and blood loss may lead to hypovolemia and decline in cardiac output. Mild hypothermia may conserve energy by reducing energy expenditure. Elevated circulating levels of insulin and counterregulatory hormones (catecholamines, glucagon, antidiuretic hormone) promote mobilization of substrates to provide for wound repair, leukocyte production, and acute phase protein synthesis. The acute injury response may last 48–72 hr., and is followed by hypermetabolism that usually peaks 3–4 days after the initial insult (22). This is a period of intense metabolic activity as indicated in Table 1-1. If the precipitating insult is not corrected or goes unrecognized, hypermetabolism persists and the organ failure syndrome may begin. In a small percentage of patients the inciting stress is sustained or severe enough to trigger progressive hypermetabolism, organ failure, and death.

Following an injury, a period of decreased cardiac output with decreased oxygen delivery occurs. Organ uptake of oxygen (VO_2) can be maintained at a constant level over a wide range of oxygen delivery (DO_2 (23) by increasing oxygen extraction from the red cells or by increasing the cross-sectional area of perfused capillaries (1). Once this recruitable oxygen reserve is exhausted, the body is no longer able to maintain the normal intracellular redox potential. When the oxygen demand of the enzyme systems of the mitochondrion exceeds delivery, glycolysis within the cytosol meets energy requirements by reducing pyruvate to lactate. It is assumed that the energy needed for cellular function and continued differentiation and maturation can be provided, albeit in a much less efficient manner.

In patients with hypermetabolism, the extraction of oxygen may be markedly abnormal (24). Oxygen consumption is dependent on oxygen delivery, so the compensatory microvascular mechanisms must be altered in such a way that an oxygen demand–supply imbalance exists due to altered blood flow distribution or direct endothelial or parenchymal injury to the organ (1). According to the altered blood flow theory, oxygenated blood bypasses nutrient capillaries, with an increased portion of the cardiac output going to organs with low oxygen extraction (e.g., skeletal muscle) or being shunted in precapillary arteriovenous channels that do not reach the cells.

There is little information available on structural changes in the enterocyte in the setting of hypermetabolism/organ failure. The low-flow state of acute injury response may disrupt normal enterocyte function with resultant compromise of structural integrity. The microscopic mucosal changes in ischemic gut injury have been examined in a canine model by Chiu et al. (25). The key factor that triggers ischemic mucosal changes has been thought to be hypoxia or decreased oxygen delivery. Vasoactive amines or oxygen radicals (26) may also have roles upon reperfusion of ischemic intestine. Mucosal lesions in humans with shock (27) have been studied and found to resemble those of animal models.

The enterocytes serve dual roles as secretors and absorbers of luminal contents as well as a barrier to intraluminal bacteria and to the loss of essential biomolecules. The invasion of bacteria across the epithelial barrier is prevented by mechanical factors including the mucin layer that rests on the epithelium and the tight junctions between cells; as well as immunologic factors such as secretory IgA, gut-associated lymphoid tissues, and mesenteric lymph nodes; and nutritive factors such as adequate blood flow. The intestinal epithelium is composed of columnar cells with intercellular spaces through which substances can flow in a paracellular or transcellular manner (Figure 1-1). The major route of nutrient flux is a paracellular one bounded on the luminal side by intercellular tight junctions. Diamond (28) has referred to this junctional complex as a physiological fence–gate–bridge system. The fence prevents diffusion of gastrointestinal contents into the body proper and the leakage of biomolecules into the gut lumen, the gate allows passive diffusion of water and small molecules between interstitium and lumen, and the bridge permits intracellular movement of essential cell messengers. The paracellular barrier can be further divided into the tight junction, also known as the zonula occludens (ZO) (29), and the underlying intercellular space. The ZO structure was first described by Farquhar and Palade (30) and recently reviewed by Gumbiner (31). The dynamics of the ZO in intestinal disease may serve to explain the central role of the gut in the systemic stress response.

Madara (29) has reviewed work suggesting that the ZO may play a pivotal

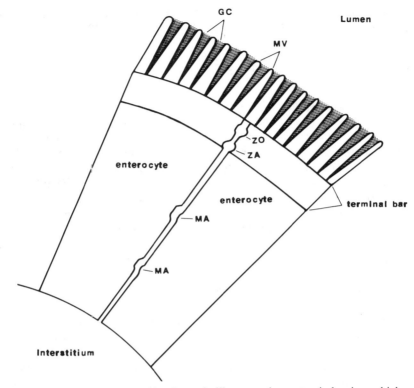

Figure 1-1. The enterocyte. A schematic illustrates the anatomic barriers which control paracellular movement of molecules.
GC—glycocalyx, MV—microvilli, ZO—zonula occludens, ZA—zonula adherens, MA—macula adherens.

role as a barrier following hypoxic stress and invasion of polymorphonuclear leukocytes (PMN). These studies have relied on the use of a model intestinal epithelium consisting of T_{84} cells (32), which are similar to native intestinal epithelium (29). Acute stress or inflammation causes the movement of PMN from the subepithelial vasculature into and across the intestinal epithelium (33). Zonula occludens function can be demonstrated to be dramatically impaired when PMN are chemically stimulated to cross a T_{84} monolayer. It appears that the PMN may actually pull the ZO apart in a mechanical fashion, allowing leakage of biomolecules and other substances previously mentioned (34). This destruction of the barrier may lead to brush border enzyme loss, intestinal villus atrophy, and mucosal edema with a decrease in intestinal absorptive capacity. Edema of the gastrointestinal tract may alter Starling forces, causing an egress of albumin and other proteins with resultant protein losing enteropathy (35). The role of enterocyte compromise in injury response is summarized in Figure 1-2.

SYSTEMIC RESPONSE TO GUT INJURY

After an acute stress, the body reacts with an acute inflammatory response characterized by local vasodilation with increased local blood flow, capillary permeability and leakage of fluid into the interstitial space, local coagulation, and cellular swelling. The inflammatory response is thought to be mediated by neutrophils and macrophages. An increase in parenchymal neutrophils is seen in models of adult respiratory distress syndrome, not only in the lungs but also in nonpulmonary organs (36). Morphologic changes associated with acute inflammation, including sequestration, degranulation, and fragmentation of neutrophils, have been demonstrated in primate models of sepsis (37). The mechanism of action seems to be an interplay between mediators released by the PMN, macrophages, injured cells, and the capillary epithelium.

The term *translocation* has been coined to describe the movement of bacteria, endotoxins, and antigenic substances across the intestinal barrier. Factors promoting this process include bacterial overgrowth (38), altered host defenses (39), and disruption of the intestinal mucosal barrier (40). The indigenous bacteria of the gastrointestinal tract are the primary source of endotoxins, which are a heterogeneous group of molecules derived from the lipopolysaccharide portion of the outer membrane of gram-negative bacteria. The tight junctions between columnar epithelium of the gastrointestinal tract normally serve as an impermeable barrier to the passage of bacteria and endotoxin, but during the injury response breakdown of barrier function allows endotoxins to enter the portal vein and intestinal lymphatics. The events that lead to translocation of endotoxin are unknown, but evidence suggests that vasoactive amines may be factors (41). The systemic effects of endotoxemia may be the result of passage of endotoxin through intestinal lymphatics since endotoxemia still occurs with ligation of the portal vein (42). Once endotoxins gain entry to the systemic circulation, there may be further loss of mucosal integrity, with a generalized increase in vasopermeability and impairment of immune function.

Injection of endotoxin into animal models (43) or human volunteers (44) produces a syndrome of fever, hypotension, tachypnea, interstitial fluid sequestration, decreased cardiac output, hypoperfusion, and metabolic acidosis, which resembles the septic injury response. Endotoxin has been shown to bind to specific receptors on the cell membrane and subcellular organelles, culminating in endothelial injury with membrane destabilization and increased vasopermeability (45, 46). It has also been shown that cultured endothelial cells release prostacyclin (PGI_2) in response to endotoxin challenge (47).

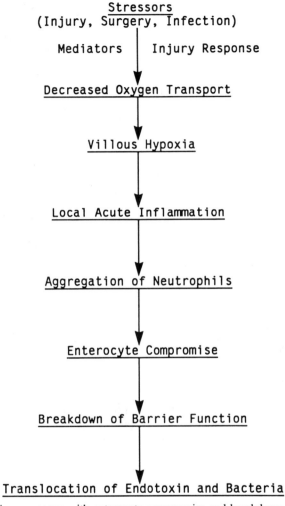

Figure 1-2. Injury response with enterocyte compromise and breakdown of gut barrier function.

Endotoxin also triggers PMN and macrophages to release a variety of stress mediators that include interleukin-1 (IL-1), granulocyte–monocyte colony-stimulating factor (GM-CSF), and tumor necrosis factor (TNF) (48). Many of the systemic effects of endotoxins are directed by these mediators. Although it is difficult to pinpoint a single mediator in injury response, it is TNF that is elevated in animal models of sepsis (49) as well as in humans with septic shock (50).

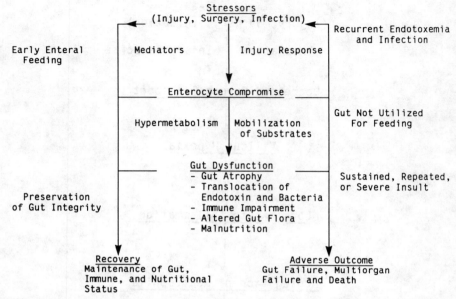

Figure 1-3. The central role of the gut in the hypermetabolic response to injury. Gut dysfunction lowers the threshold for adverse outcome, with gut atrophy, translocation of endotoxin and bacteria, immune impairment, altered gut flora, and malnutrition, all favoring continued injury response and unchecked hypermetabolism.

Tumor necrosis factor has a host of metabolic, vascular, and immune effects that may account for many of the unfortunate sequelae of sepsis. Monoclonal antibody to TNF has been shown to be protective in a lethal animal model of bacterial sepsis (51). The degree of elevation of TNF levels may also correlate with death due to sepsis in critically ill humans (50).

CONCLUSION

The gut has a paramount role in the mediation of injury response because translocation of endotoxin across a disrupted gut barrier may be one of triggering events of the multiorgan failure syndrome (Figure 1-3). The consequent release of stress mediators including cytokines, eicosanoids, and neuroendocrine factors will have an adverse impact on a variety of gut functions and favor continued injury response and unchecked hypermetabolism.

In addition to mediator and barrier functions, the gut is a metabolically active organ that utilizes and processes multiple substrates. A variety of nutrients are being studied for their role in maintaining optimal gut function. Nutrients that are not otherwise limiting may be conditionally essential in the setting of hypermetabolism and injury. These will be reviewed elsewhere in this text and include amino acids, nucleic acids, and alternative fat substrates. Although the optimal diet composition to maintain favorable gut function remains unclear, there is a growing body of information to support the use of enteral feeding whenever possible. Enteral feeding is the preferred and physiological route to supply nutrition in malnourished patients. It appears to maintain a functional intestinal mucosa with improved nutrient utilization and protection against translocation of bacteria, endotoxins, and antigenic substances. Enteral feeding should be given a high priority in the injured patient because disruption of intestinal barrier function may promote hypermetabolism and multiple organ failure.

REFERENCES

1. Dorinsky, PM, Cadek JE: Mechanisms of multiple nonpulmonary organ failure in ARDS. Chest 96:885, 1989.
2. Madara, JL, Trier JS: Functional morphology of the mucosa of the small intestine, in Johnson LR (ed) Physiology of the Gastrointestinal Tract, Second edition. New York, Raven Press, 1987.
3. Eastwood GL: Small bowel morphology and epithelial proliferation in intravenously alimented rabbits. Surgery 82:613, 1977.
4. Levine GM, Denen JJ, Steiger ET, et al: Role of oral intake in maintenance of gut mass and disaccharide activity. Gastroenterology 67:975, 1974.
5. Feldman EJ, Dowling RH, McNaughton J, et al: Effects of oral versus intravenous nutrition on intestinal adaptation after small bowel resection in the dog. Gastroenterology 70:712, 1976.
6. Ford WDA, Boelhauwer RU, Kind WWK, et al: total parenteral nutrition inhibits intestinal adaptive hyperplasia in rabbits. Reversal by feeding. Surgery 96:527, 1984.
7. Straggard JJ, Hagemann RF: Effect of luminal contents on colonic cell replacement. Am J Physiol 233:E208, 1977.
8. Maxton DG, Cynk EU, Thompson RPH: Small intestinal response to "elemental" and "complete" liquid feeds in the rat: effect of dietary bulk. Gut 28:688, 1987.
9. Altmann GG: Influence of bile and pancreatic secretions on the size of the intestinal villi in the rat. Am J Anat 132:167, 1971.
10. Williamson RCN: Intestinal adaptation (Part 2): mechanisms of control. N Engl J Med 298:1444, 1978.
11. Williamson RCN, Bauer FLR, Ross JS, et al: Contributions of bile and of pancreatic juice to cell proliferation in ileal mucosa. Surgery 83:570, 1978.
12. Loran MR, Cracker IT: Population dynamics of intestinal epithelia in the rat two months after partial resection of the ileum. J Cell Biol 19:285, 1963.

13. Johnson IR: The trophic action of gastrointestinal hormones. Gastroenterology 70:278, 1976.
14. Gleeson MH, Bloom SR, Polak, JM, et al: Endocrine tumor in kidney affecting small bowel structure, motility, and absorptive function. Gut 12:773, 1971.
15. Tilson MD, Phillips S, Wright HK: An effect of deoxycorticosteroid upon the ileum stimulating compensatory hypertrophy of the gut. Surgery 69:730, 1971.
16. Taylor B, Murphy GM, Dowling RH: Effect of food intake and the pituitary on intestinal structure and function after small bowel resection in the rat. Gut 16:397, 1975.
17. Wright NA, Marley AR, Appleton D: The effect of testosterone on cell proliferation and differentiation in the small bowel. J Endocrinol 52:161, 1972.
18. Tutton PJM: Neural and endocrine control systems acting on the population kinetics of the intestinal epithelium. Med Biol 55:201, 1977.
19. Sagor GR, Ghatei MA, Al-Mukhtar MYT, et al: Evidence for a humoral mechanism after small bowel resection. Exclusion of gastrin but not enteroglucagon. Gastroenterology 84:902, 1983.
20. Cuthbertson DP: The disturbance of metabolism produced by bony and non-bony injury with notes on certain abnormal conditions of bone. Biochem J 24:1244, 1930.
21. Cuthbertson DP: Observations on the disturbances of metabolism produced by injury to the limbs. Q J Med 1:233, 1932.
22. Cerra FG: Hypermetabolism, organ failure, and metabolic support. Surgery 101:1, 1987.
23. Cain SM: Assessment of tissue oxygenation. Crit Care Clin 2:537, 1986.
24. Danek SJ, Lynch JP, Weg JG, et al: The dependence of oxygen uptake on oxygen delivery in the adult respiratory distress syndrome. Am Rev Respir Dis 122:387, 1980.
25. Chiu CJ, McArdle AH, Brown R, et al: Intestinal mucosal lesion in low-flow states. Arch Surg 101:478, 1970.
26. Parks DA, Bulkley GB, Granger DN, et al: Ischemic injury in the cat small intestine: role of superoxide radicals. Gastroenterology 82:9, 1982.
27. Haglund U, Hulten L, Ahren C, et al: Mucosal lesions in the human small intestine in shock. Gut 16:979, 1975.
28. Diamond JM: The epithelial junction: bridge, gate, and fence. Physiologist 20:10, 1977.
29. Madara JL: Loosening tight junctions: lessons from the intestine. J Clin Invest 83:1089, 1989.
30. Farquhar MG, Palade GE: Junctional complexes in various epithelia. J. Cell Biol. 17:375, 1963.
31. Gumbiner B: The structure, biochemistry, and assembly of epithelial tight junctions. Am J Physiol 253:C749, 1987.

32. Dharmsathaphorn K, Mandel KG, McRoberts JA, et al: A human colonic tumor cell line that maintains vectorial electrolyte transport. Am J Physiol 246:G204, 1984.
33. Kumar NB, Nostrant TT, Appleman HD: The histopathologic spectrum of acute self-limited colitis (acute infectious-type colitis). Am J Surg Pathol 6:523, 1982.
34. Nash S, Stafford J, Madara JL: The selective and superoxide-independent disruption of intestinal epithelial tight junctions during leukocyte transmigration. Lab Invest 59:531, 1988.
35. Brinson RR, Pitts WM: Gastrointestinal complications of acute respiratory failure: analogy between adult respiratory distress syndrome, gastrointestinal edema, and enteral feeding intolerance. Crit Care Med 17:841, 1989.
36. Mizer L, Weisbrode S, Dorinsky PM: Neutrophil accumulation and structural changes in non-pulmonary organs following phorbol myristate acetete-induced lung injury. Am Rev Respir Dis 139:1017, 1989.
37. Coalson JJ, Hinshaw LB, Guenter CA, et al: Pathophysiologic responses of the subhuman primate in experimental septic shock. Lab Invest 32:561, 1975.
38. Deitch EA, Maejima K, Berg R: Effect of oral antibiotics and bacterial overgrowth on the translocation of the GI tract microflora in burned rats. J Trauma 25:385, 1985.
39. Deitch EA, Winterton J, Berg R: Deficiency of T cell-mediated immunity promotes bacterial translocation from the GI tract after thermal injury. Arch Surg 121:97, 1986.
40. Li M, Specian RD, Berg R, et al: Effects of protein malnutrition and endotoxin on the intestinal mucosal barrier to the translocation of indigenous flora in mice. JPEN 13:572, 1989.
41. Cuevas P, Fine J: Production of fatal endotoxin shock by vasoactive substances. Gastroenterology 64:285, 1973.
42. Olcay I, Katahama A, Miller RH, et al: Reticuloendothelial dysfunction and endotoxemia following portal vein occlusion. Surgery 75:64, 1974.
43. Natanson C, Eichenholz PW, Danner RL, et al: Endotoxin and tumor necrosis factor challenges in dogs stimulate the cardiovascular profile of human septic shock. J. Exp Med 169:823, 1989.
44. Suffredini AF, Fromm RE, Praker MM, et al: The Cardiovascular response of normal humans to the administration of endotoxin. N Engl J Med 521:280, 1989.
45. Morrison DC, Rudbach JA: Endotoxin–cell membrane interactions leading to transmembrane signaling. Contemp Top Mol Immunol 8:187, 1981.
46. Watson J, Kelly K, Whitlock C: Genetic control of endotoxin sensitivity, in Schlesinger D (ed) Microbiology—1980. Washington, DC: American Society of Microbiology, 1980.
47. Rossi V, Breviario F, Ghezzi P, et al: Interleukin-1 induced prostacyclin in vascular cells. Science 229:1174, 1985.

48. Jacobs RF, Tabor DR: Immune cellular interactions during sepsis and septic injury. Crit Care Clin 5:9, 1989.
49. Grunfeld C, Palladino MA: Tumor necrosis factor: immunologic, antitumor, metabolic, and cardiovascular activities. Adv Intern Med 55:45, 1990.
50. Debets JMH, Kampmeijer R, Van Der Linden MP, et al: Plasma tumor necrosis factor and mortality in critically ill septic patients. Crit Care Med 17:489, 1989.
51. Tracey KJ, Fong Y, Hesse DG, et al: Anti-cachectin/TNF monoclonal antibodies prevent septic shock during lethal bacteremia. Nature 330:662, 1987.

Bacterial Translocation

CHAPTER 2

Jason G. Nirgiotis, M.D.
and Richard J. Andrassy, M.D., F.A.C.S.

INTRODUCTION

Sepsis is a frequent cause of morbidity and mortality in critically ill patients. Sepsis may result in multiple organ failure, which often leads to death. One theory of the cause of sepsis in severely ill patients is that bacteria normally confined within the gastrointestinal tract are the source of the infection. These bacteria cross the intestinal mucosal barrier and invade the lymph nodes and other organs in a process called bacterial translocation (1). It is believed that this occurs when a motile phagocyte ingests bacteria, transports them to extraintestinal tissues, fails to kill them, and then releases the bacteria (2).

The gut is directly connected to the outside world and contains large amounts of bacteria and endotoxin. It has been recognized that under normal circumstances the intestinal mucosa prevents bacteria that colonize the gut from invading systemic organs and tissues. Certainly damage to the outside skin barrier (i.e., burn injury) allows bacteria to colonize the tissue and leads to infection and hypermetabolism. It appears that under certain circumstances the gut can serve as a reservoir for bacteria that cause systemic infections. Growing evidence suggests that many of the infections we see in our critically ill patients (particularly immunocompromised patients) come from bacteria normally found within the gut (3). Secondary infections after severe trauma or operative intervention may be a result of this bacterial translocation (4). Certain clinical conditions such as necrotizing enterocolitis most probably occur secondary to ischemic mucosal damage and secondary bacterial translocation.

One or more of three basic pathophysiological factors are usually necessary for bacterial translocation to occur (5). These are physical disruption of the gut mucosal barrier, alteration of the normal intestinal microflora with bacterial overgrowth, and impaired host immune defenses. We will discuss the role of each of these factors in causing bacterial translocation and possible methods for preventing translocation.

DISRUPTION OF THE GUT MUCOSAL BARRIER

Sepsis frequently leads to multiple organ failure and death, but in up to 30% of patients subject to this no septic focus can be found either clinically or at autopsy (6). Since these patients are often infected with bacteria that are normally found in the intestinal lumen, it is possible that the gut may be the source of these septic episodes. Because sepsis and multiple organ failure are common in trauma victims with shock, Deitch et al. studied the link between hemorrhagic shock and bacterial translocation from the gut. In a rat model, they demonstrated that the degree of histologic intestinal damage increased with longer durations of shock (7). After 30 min of shock, there were areas of submucosal edema at the tip of the ileal villi and by 60 min the edema had increased and there were occasional focal areas of ileal mucosal necrosis. There was extensive ileal mucosal necrosis after 90 min of shock. Previous studies have shown that simple mechanical disruption of the intestinal mucosa promotes bacterial translocation (8). In the shocked rat model there was a significant increase in the number of organs and lymph nodes that contained bacteria after increasing lengths of time of shock. Rats subjected to 90 min of shock had a significantly greater degree of translocation than rats receiving 30 or 60 min of shock. The number of bacteria per gram of lymph node were increased as well (9). The 24-hr mortality rate of the animals increased proportionally to the duration of shock. *E. coli* and *Enterococcus* were the most common bacteria found to translocate.

Rush et al. have demonstrated that by the third day after shock almost all of the animals had enteric bacteremia (10). By feeding the rats radiolabeled *E. coli*, they were able to show that the *E. coli* crossed the intestinal mucosal barrier during shock and appeared in the bloodstream (11). In human studies they found that normotensive adult patients had only a 4% incidence of positive blood cultures within 3 hr of admission, but the patients with a systolic blood pressure below 80 mm Hg had a 56% incidence of positive blood cultures (12).

In further studies by Deitch's group, it was shown that bacterial translocation after hemorrhagic shock is mediated, at least in part, by xanthine oxidase-derived oxidants (13). Allopurinol, a competitive inhibitor of xanthine oxidase, decreased shock-induced bacterial translocation from 61 to 14%. In addition, translocation was reduced to 10% when xanthine oxidase was inactivated by feeding the rats a tungsten-supplemented molybdenum-free diet.

Deitch and co-workers have performed a number of other studies to clarify which factors may increase the risk of bacterial translocation. They have demonstrated that endotoxin given either intramuscularly or intraperitoneally promotes bacterial translocation in a dosage-dependent fashion from the gut to the mesenteric lymph nodes (14). This endotoxin-induced translocation is short-lived, and by 48 hr after endotoxin administration the levels and incidence of translocation had decreased. The degree of translocation and the extent of endotoxin-induced ileal mucosal injury were both reduced by inhibition or inactivation of xanthine dehydrogenase and oxidase activity (15). Endotoxin injured primarily the ileal and cecal mucosa and increased ileal and hepatic xanthine dehydrogenase and cecal oxidase activities (16). It appears from these results that xanthine oxidase-induced mucosal damage plays a role in endotoxin-induced bacterial translocation.

Ma and co-workers have used a murine burn model to demonstrate a thermally induced gut mucosal injury that led to an increase in bacterial translocation (17). Alexander and colleagues have shown in the burned animal model that blood is shunted away from the delicate mucosal lining of the gastrointestinal track (18). This leads to atrophy or damage that facilitates bacterial translocation. Hypermetabolic mediators are released secondary to this translocation, which leads to an increase in catabolism as well as increased protein and caloric requirements.

Ziegler et al. have demonstrated increased lactulose excretion in the urine of septic burned patients given oral lactulose (19). They concluded that the sepsis may be secondary to increased intestinal permeability and thus the septic burn patient may have increased bacterial translocation. Other patients who are at an increased risk for bacterial translocation due to a disruption in the gut mucosal barrier include patients with Crohn's disease (20) or radiation injury to the bowel (21).

ALTERATION OF INTESTINAL MICROFLORA

It has been shown that altering the normal intestinal microflora by allowing overgrowth of certain bacteria (especially enteric bacilli) promotes bacterial translocation (22). Burned rats given low-dosage oral penicillin had a much greater incidence of bacterial translocation than rats not given antibiotics. At the dosages given, penicillin selectively inhibited the growth of certain strictly anaerobic bacteria, thereby allowing overgrowth of other facultatively anaerobic bacteria such as *E. coli*. Gram-negative enteric bacilli, such as *E. coli, Proteus,* and *Enterobacter,* translocate at higher rates than either gram-positive or obligate anaerobic bacteria (23). When the gastrointestinal tract microflora are altered, enteric bacteria translocate to the mesenteric lymph nodes, liver, spleen, and, less commonly, the peritoneal cavity, lung, and bloodstream.

If bacterial overgrowth occurs in the intestines, greater numbers of bacteria can translocate to the lymph nodes. Deitch et al. showed that replacing the normal intestinal microflora of mice with *E. coli* not only led to a higher incidence and magnitude of translocation but also caused an increase in mortality (24). They have also demonstrated that the administration of nonlethal dosages of endotoxin disrupts the normal ecology of the gut flora, resulting in overgrowth of enteric bacilli and translocation (25).

In a clinical study of patients undergoing laparotomy, Deitch showed that simple intestinal obstruction of the colon or small bowel in the absence of necrotic bowel was associated with bacterial translocation (26). He then performed animal studies that demonstrated that bacteria had translocated to the lymph nodes within 6 hr of intestinal ligation, and to the liver, spleen, and bloodstream within 24 hr (27). It appears that bacterial translocation induced by intestinal obstruction is due to disruption of the ecology of the normal gut microflora, leading to overgrowth of certain enteric bacilli and mucosal damage.

Since bile is important in binding endotoxin, Deitch's group also studied the role of obstructive jaundice in bacterial translocation (28). Animals that underwent bile duct ligation had significantly increased levels of cecal gram-negative, enteric bacilli, and subepithelial edema involving the ileal villi. This resulted in a much greater incidence of bacterial translocation.

IMPAIRED IMMUNE DEFENSES

There is an increased risk of infection resulting from bacterial translocation in patients with impaired immune systems (29). Patients with hematologic malignancies, especially those receiving chemotherapy, have a higher incidence of infections caused by bacteria that are normally within their gastrointestinal tracts (30). A study of mice immunocompromised with cyclophosphamide demonstrated that only the alteration of normal bacterial flora was necessary for translocation of *E. coli*, but immunosuppression was needed for translocation of *P. aeruginosa* (31). Impaired host immune defenses, such as a deficiency in T-cell-mediated immunity, have been shown to promote bacterial translocation (32).

Simple protein–calorie malnutrition impairs the immune system (33,34). Protein–calorie malnutrition adversely affects more or less all immune competent cells (35). Protein malnutrition results in severe ileal atrophy and studies demonstrated that although malnutrition itself did not promote bacterial translocation, the malnourished mice were more susceptible to endotoxin-induced translocation than normally nourished mice (36). The mortality rate in the animals was directly related to the severity of malnutrition (37).

Secretory IgA is the principal immunoglobulin in the lumen of the gastrointestinal tract. It can prevent the binding of enterotoxins and microorganisms to the intestinal microvilli and block the uptake of enteric antigens (38). Thus, a decrease in the level of secretory IgA in the intestine could lead to an increased risk of bacterial translocation (39). Alverdy and colleagues have shown that rats fed enterally maintained secretory IgA levels better than rats fed the same nutrients intravenously (40). They have also shown that rats fed standard total parenteral nutrition (TPN) for 2 weeks had a 66% incidence of positive cultures in mesenteric lymph nodes. None of the animals fed standard rat chow had evidence of bacterial translocation (41).

After trauma or hemorrhagic shock, there is decreased neutrophil chemotaxis and phagocytosis and a reversal of the T-cell helper to suppressor ratio (42). These factors may play a role in the increased bacterial translocation seen following trauma and shock (11). It has also been shown that immunosuppression with prednisone or cyclophosphamide accelerates the translocation that occurs with bacterial overgrowth (43). Thus, it appears that an impaired immune system is a predisposing factor to bacterial translocation.

PREVENTING BACTERIAL TRANSLOCATION

Major causative factors in bacterial translocation include a disruption in the mucosal barrier, bacterial overgrowth, and an impaired immune system. Therefore, the rate of translocation might be decreased if the gastrointestinal tract integrity could be protected, normal bacterial flora preserved, or the immune system improved in critically ill patients.

Several specific micronutrients have recently been shown to stimulate the immune system and therefore might be of benefit in decreasing the incidence of bacterial translocation. Glutamine has been shown to be protective of the gastrointestinal mucosa in a number of conditions (44) and with certain treatment modalities, such as chemotherapy (45) or radiotherapy (46). Burke et al. demonstrated that glutamine-supplemented total parenteral nutrition improves immune function by decreasing the incidence of bacterial translocation and preventing the decrease in secretory IgA usually seen with total parenteral nutrition (47). Several studies have shown that supplemental arginine improves host immune defenses (48). Studies in our own laboratories with young rats have shown that arginine-supplemented animals had significantly enhanced immune responses, as demonstrated by significantly increased lymphocyte activation and blastogenesis of lymphocytes when cultured with the mitogens phytohemagglutinin (PHA) and concanavalin A (Con A) (49). In addition, the arginine-supplemented group lived significantly longer following bacterial challenge than did the arginine-free group. Glutamine and arginine is discussed in greater detail in Chapter 5.

Since gram-negative enteric bacilli appear to be the bacteria that translocate most often, several groups have attempted to decrease the incidence of systemic infections in critically ill patients by selectively decontaminating the gut with oral nonabsorbable antibiotics directed against gram-negative bacilli. When combined with topical hypopharyngeal antibiotics, selective gut decontamination decreases the incidence of systemic infections in both intensive care unit patients and trauma victims (50,51).

In patients with granulocytopenia and patients with cancer, selective gut decontamination produces a lower rate of gram-negative enteric bacteremia than occurs in conventionally treated patients (52). However, this treatment remains controversial since there is no difference in survival rates with or without decontamination.

Studies by Andrassy and co-workers have shown the value of enteral feeding in protecting the intestinal mucosa from stress ulcers and mucosal damage (53,54). Saito et al. demonstrated in guinea pigs that enteral diets provided better nutrition, maintained gut mucosal integirty better, and prevented an increased secretion of catabolic hormones compared to total parenteral nutrition (55). Direct stimulation of the gut-associated lymphoid tissue by enteral feedings has been demonstrated in both animal and human models (39,56). Several studies have demonstrated enteral nutrition to be superior to the TPN in maintaining the gut's immunologic function (57–59). Thus it appears that the type of nutrients given and the method of feeding are critical to maintaining a normal gastrointestinal tract and preventing bacterial translocation (60).

CONCLUSION

What is the clinical significance of bacterial translocation? It is evident that bacteremia itself is not necessarily harmful. Episodes of bacteremia frequently occur in healthy patients after colonoscopy and brushing teeth, with no ill effects (61,62). Simple laparotomy with minimal bowel manipulation causes bacterial translocation and bacteremia (63). It appears that only in patients who are compromised in some way might these transient episodes of bacteremia lead to sepsis. Patients with trauma that have injured several organ systems or who have had an episode of hypotension seem to be more susceptible to sepsis. These patients and others who have an impaired immune system for a variety of reasons are less able to combat bacteremia. From the available evidence it seems that it is this subgroup of patients that is most likely to experience sepsis following an episode of bacterial translocation. Therefore efforts must be made to find better ways to decrease the incidence of translocation in these ill patients by protecting the mucosal barrier or improving the immune system.

REFERENCES

1. Berg RD, Garlington AW: Translocation of certain indigenous bacteria from the gastrointestinal tract to the mesenteric lymph nodes and other organs in a gnobiotic mouse model. Infect Immun 23:403–411, 1979.
2. Wells CL, Maddaus MA, Simmons RL: Proposed mechanisms for the translocation of intestinal bacteria. Rev Infect Dis 10:958–979, 1988.
3. Andrassy RJ: Preserving the gut mucosal barrier and enhancing immune response. Contemp Surg 32:1–7, 1988.
4. Page CP: The surgeon and gut maintenance. Am J Surg 158:485–490, 1989.
5. Deitch EA: The role of intestinal barrier failure and bacterial translocation in the development of systemic infection and multiple organ failure. Arch Surg 125:403–404, 1990.
6. Carrico CJ, Meakins JL, Marshall JC, et al: Multiple organ failure syndrome. Arch Surg 121:196–208, 1986.
7. Baker JW, Deitch EA, Li M, et al: Hemorrhagic shock induces bacterial translocation from the gut. J Trauma 28:896–906, 1988.
8. Morehouse J, Specian R, Stewart J, et al: Promotion of the translocation of indigenous bacteria of mice from the G.I. tract by oral ricinoleic acid. Gastroenterology 91:673–682, 1986.
9. Deitch EA, Bridges RM: Effect of stress and trauma in bacterial translocation from the gut. J Surg Res 42:536–542, 1987.
10. Koziol J, Rush B, Smith S, et al: Occurrence of bacteremia during and after hemorrhagic shock. J Trauma 28:10–15, 1988.
11. Sori A, Rush B, Lysz T, et al: The gut as a source of sepsis following hemorrhagic shock. Am J Surg 155:187–192, 1988.
12. Rush BF, Sori AJ, Murphy TF, et al: Endotoxemia and bacteremia during hemorrhagic shock. The link between trauma and sepsis? Ann Surg 207:549–554, 1988.
13. Deitch EA, Bridges W, Baker J, et al: Hemorrhagic shock-induced bacterial translocation is reduced by xanthine oxidase inhibition or inactivation. Surgery 104:191–198, 1988.
14. Deitch EA, Berg R, Specian R: Endotoxin promotes the translocation of bacteria from the gut. Arch Surg 122:185–190, 1987.
15. Deitch EA, Ma L, Jing W, et al: Inhibition of endotoxin-induced bacterial translocation in mice. J Clin Invest 84:36–42, 1989.

16. Deitch EA, Taylor M, Grisham M, et al: Endotoxin induces bacterial translocation and increases xanthine oxidase activity. J Trauma 29:1679–1683, 1989.
17. Ma L, Ma JW, Deitch EA, et al: Genetic susceptibility to mucosal damage leads to bacterial translocation in a murine burn model. J Trauma 29:1245–1251, 1989.
18. Alexander JW: Nutrition and infection. New perspectives for an old problem. Arch Surg 121:966–972, 1986.
19. Ziegler TR, Smith RJ, O'Dwyer ST, et al: Increased intestinal permeability associated with infection in burn patients. Arch Surg 123:1313–1319, 1988.
20. Ambrose NS, Johnson M, Burdon DW, et al: Incidence of pathogenic bacteria from mesenteric lymph nodes and ileal serosa during Crohn's disease surgery. Br J Surg 71:623–625, 1984.
21. Guzman-Stein G, Bonsack M, Liberty J, et al: Abdominal radiation causes bacterial translocation. J Surg Res 46:104–107, 1989.
22. Deitch EA, Maejuma K, Berg R: Effect of oral antibiotics and bacterial overgrowth on the translocation of the G.I. tract microflora in burned rats. J Trauma 25:385–392, 1985.
23. Steffan EK, Berg RD, Deitch EA: Comparison of translocation rates of various indigenous bacteria from the gastrointestinal tract to the mesenteric lymph node. J Infec Dis 157:1032–1038, 1988.
24. Deitch EA, Ma L, Ma WJ, et al: Lethal burn-induced bacterial translocation: role of genetic resistance. J Trauma 29:1480–1487, 1989.
25. Deitch EA, Ma WJ, Ma L, et al: Endotoxin-induced bacterial tarnslocation: a study of mechanisms. Surgery 106:292–300, 1989.
26. Deitch EA: Simple intestinal obstruction causes bacterial translocation in man. Arch Surg 124:699–701, 1989.
27. Deitch EA, Bridges WM, Ma JW, et al: Obstructed intestine as a reservoir for systemic infection. Am J Surg 159:394–401, 1990.
28. Deitch EA, Sittig K, Li M, et al: Obstructive jaundice promotes bacterial translocation from the gut. Am J Surg 159:79–84, 1990.
29. Deitch DA: The immunocompromised host. Surg Clin North Am 68:181–190, 1988.
30. Tancrede CH, Andremont AO: Bacterial translocation and gram-negative bacteremia in patients with hematological malignancies. J Infec Dis 152:99–103, 1985.
31. Tomomo K: Etiology of sepsis occurring in the immunocompromised host and its prevention. 1. Analysis of the bacterial portal of entrance in experimental mice with bacteremia. Kansenshogaku Zasshi 63:479–488, 1989.
32. Deitch EA, Winerton J, Berg R: Deficiency of T-cell mediated immunity promotes bacterial translocation from the G.I. tract after thermal injury. Arch Surg 121:97–101, 1986.
33. Chandra RK: Malnutrition, in Chandra RK (ed) Primary and Secondary Immunodeficiency Disorders. New York: Churchill Livingstone, 1983, pp. 187–203.
34. Chandra RK: Rosette-forming T-lymphocytes and cell-mediated immunity in malnutrition. Br Med J 3:608–609, 1974.

35. Garre MA, Boles JM, Yovinou PY: Current concepts in immune derangement due to undernutrition. JPEN 11:309–313, 1987.
36. Li M, Specian RD, Berg RD, et al: Effects of protein malnutrition and endotoxin on the intestinal mucosal barrier to the translocation of indigenous flora in mice. JPEN 13:572–578, 1989.
37. Deitch EA, Winterton J, Berg R: The gut as a portal of entry for bacteremia: the role of protein malnutrition. Ann Surg 205:681–692, 1987.
38. Andre C, Lambert R, Bazin H, et al: Interference of oral immunization with the intestinal absorption of heterologous albumin. Eur J Immunol 4:701–704, 1974.
39. Alverdy JC: The GI tract as an immunologic organ. Contemp Surg 35(suppl):14–19, 1989.
40. Alverdy J, Chi HS, Sheldon GF: The effect of parenteral nutrition on gastrointestinal immunity: the importance of enteral stimulation. Ann Surg 202:681–684, 1985.
41. Alverdy J, Aoys E, Moss G: Total parenteral nutrition promotes bacterial translocation from the gut. Surgery 104:185–190, 1988.
42. Christou NV, McLean APH, Meakins JL: Host defense in blunt trauma: interrelationships of kinetics of anergy and depressed neutrophil function, nutritional status and sepsis. J Trauma 20:833–841, 1980.
43. Berg RD, Wommack E, Deitch EA: Immunosuppression and intestinal bacterial overgrowth synergistically promote bacterial translocation. Arch Surg 123:1359–1364, 1988.
44. O'Dwyer ST, Smith RJ, Hwang TL et al: Maintenance of small bowel mucosa with glutamine-enriched parenteral nutrition. JPEN 13:579–585, 1989.
45. Fox AD, Kripke SA, De Paula J, et al: Effect of a glutamine-supplemented enteral diet on methotrexate-induced enterocolitis. JPEN 12:325–331, 1988.
46. Souba WW, Klimberg VS, Hautamaki RD, et al: Oral glutamine reduces bacterial translocation following abdominal radiation. J Surg Res 48:1–5, 1990.
47. Burke DJ, Alberdy JC, Aoys E, et al: Glutamine-supplemented total parenteral nutrition improves gut immune function. Arch Surg 124:1396–1399, 1989.
48. Barbul A: Arginine and immune function. Nutrition 6:53–58, 1990.
49. Nirgiotis JG, Andrassy RJ, Hennessey PJ: The effects of an arginine-free enteral diet upon wound healing and immune function in the post-surgical rat. J Pediatr Surg (in press).
50. Stoutenbeek CP, van Saene HK, Miranda DR, et al: The prevention of superinfection in multiple trauma patients. J Antimicrob Chemother 14 (suppl B):203–211, 1984.
51. Stoutenbeek CP, van Saene HK, Zandstra DF: The effect of oral non-absorbable antibiotics on the emergence of resistant bacteria in patients in an intensive care unit. J Antimicrob Chemother 19:513–520, 1987.
52. De Pauw BE, Novakova IR, Ubachs E, et al: Co-trimoxazole in patients with haematological malignancies: a review of 10-years' clinical experience. Curr Med Res Opin 11:54–72, 1988.

53. Mabogunje OA, Andrassy RJ, Isaacs H, et al: The role of a defined formula diet in the prevention of stress-induced gastric mucosal injury in the rat. J Pediatr Surg 16:1036–1038, 1981.
54. Lally KP, Andrassy RJ, Foster JE, et al: Evaluation of various nutritional supplements in the prevention of stress-induced gastric ulcers in the rat. Surg Gyn Obstet 158:124–127, 1984.
55. Saito H, Trocki O, Alexander JW, et al: The effect of route of nutrient administration on the nutritional state, metabolic hormone secretion and gut mucosal integrity following burn injury. JPEN 11:1–7, 1987.
56. Kudsk KA, Stone JM, Carpenter G, et al: Enteral and parenteral feeding influences mortality after hemoglobin-*E. coli* peritonitis in normal rats. J Trauma 23:605–609, 1983.
57. Kudsk KA, Carpenter G, Petersen SR, et al: Effect of enteral and parenteral feeding in malnourished rats with hemoglobin-*E. coli* adjuvant peritonitis. J Surg Res 31:105–110, 1981.
58. Birkhahn RH, Renk CM: Immune response and leucine oxidation in oral and intravenous fed rats. Am J Clin Nutr 39:45–53, 1984.
59. Moore FA, Moore EE, Jones TN, et al: TEN versus TPN following major abdominal trauma—reduced septic morbidity. J Trauma 29:916–923, 1989.
60. Andrassy RJ: Practical rewards of enteral feeding for the surgical patient. Contemp. Surg 35 (Suppl):20–24, 1989.
61. Low DE, Shoenut JP, Kennedy JK, et al: Prospective assessment of risk of bacteremia with colonoscopy and polypectomy. Dig Dis Sci 32:1239–1243, 1987.
62. Silver JG, Martin AW, McBride BC: Experimental transient bacteremias in human subjects with clinically healthy gingivae. J Clin Peridontol 6:33–36, 1979.
63. Redan JA, Rush BF Jr, Lysz TW, et al: Organ distribution of gut-derived bacteria caused by bowel manipulation or ischemia. Am J Surg 159:85–90, 1990.

Enteral Nutrition and Critical Illness

CHAPTER 3

John L. Rombeau, M.D.

INTRODUCTION

Continued advances in the monitoring and support of vital organ systems have led to increased survival of patients with life-threatening conditions such as overwhelming sepsis and acute episodes of respiratory, cardiac, renal, and hepatic failure. The administration of either enteral or parenteral feeding (nutritional support) is now an integral part of the therapy of malnourished hospitalized patients. However, the need for these feedings in critically ill patients is often unclear. Many critically ill patients are either too ill or their life expectancy is too short to permit the initiation of nutritional support. Other critical ill patients are subject to so many forms of invasive monitoring and therapy that nutritional intervention becomes a low priority. The advent and widespread use of parenteral nutrition have demonstrated that the nutritional status of these patients can be supported temporarily until the critical illness subsides (1).

Recent research indicates that the gastrointestinal (GI) tract participates in the body's response to stress and may become the source of sepsis and multiple organ system failure syndrome (MOFs) (2). Although the provision of nutrients may attenuate the deleterious effects of stress on the GI tract, critical illnesses are commonly associated with GI disorders that make it difficult, if not impossible, to administer enteral nutrition (EN). To determine the need for and feasibility of providing EN to critically ill patients, it is essential to understand the pathophysiology of the GI tract during critical illnesses. This chapter reviews this topic and describes the indications for administering EN to critically ill patients. This information has been excerpted from a previous publication on this topic (3).

EFFECTS OF STRESS ON THE GASTROINTESTINAL TRACT

Since the advent of parenteral nutrition, it has not been essential to have a functioning GI tract to survive critical illnesses. Therefore, less attention has been devoted to developing techniques for monitoring the GI tract in the intensive care unit (ICU). As a consequence, the GI response to critical illnesses is poorly understood. Nevertheless, it is evident that the GI mucosa is susceptible to ulceration and bleeding and to ischemia during stress (4).

Despite the absence of a specific injury to the GI tract, ileus commonly occurs in critically ill patients. In these patients, ileus may result from either the primary disease or its treatment. Ileus, most commonly referred to as paralytic ileus, may be due to many different causes and each of these may act singularly or in combination (5). Abdominal surgery (apart from GI procedures) is a frequent cause of ileus in patients admitted to the ICU. The cause of postoperative ileus is still not well understood, and it is probably due to many factors, including reflex alpha-sympathetic stimulation, peritonitis, hypokalemia, intraperitoneal hemorrhage, and spillage of enteric fluids (6). Other clinical conditions associated with paralytic ileus include intra-abdominal sepsis, intrathoracic or retroperitoneal disease, intestinal ischemia, head and spinal injuries, metabolic disorders (uremia, diabetic coma, and myxedema), and administration of ganglionic blocking agents.

The various segments of the gut are unequally susceptible to paralytic ileus. The small bowel is somewhat resistant to the development of ileus, and motility and absorption capacity usually returns within the first 24 hr following insult. The colon and stomach may take 3 or more days to recover normal motility after intra-abdominal surgery. In addition, gastric motility is impaired by numerous drugs given in the ICU, such as anticholinergic agents, beta-adrenergic antagonists, calcium channel blockers, and dopamine antagonists.

One of the features of ileus is the loss of the interdigestive motor complex (IMC). This normal motion pattern of the intestine prevents stagnation of bacteria in the small bowel. Loss of the interdigestive motor complex is associated with bacterial overgrowth of the small intestine (7). Stagnation of bacteria, particularly in the colon, has been implicated as a predisposing factor in the development of *Clostridium difficile*—induced diarrhea (8).

THE GASTROINTESTINAL TRACT AS A SOURCE OF STRESS

Since the widespread use of broad-spectrum antibiotics, the incidence and mortality of infection due to exogenous bacteria have declined, but a sharp rise has occurred in the incidence of infections caused by endogenous bacteria. In the 1960s, gram-negative bacteria were the leading cause of infection in hospitalized patients. More recently, a group of organisms of obscure origin and uncertain pathogenicity, including the enterococci, *Staphylococcus epidermidis*, and *Candida*, have been recognized as common infecting agents in critically ill patients (2). The prevalence of MOFS has increased concurrently with this shift in the epidemiology of infection and improvements in supportive care. Bacteremia and endotoxemia are most likely associated with this syndrome, although a consistent correlation with positive blood cultures and identifiable bacterial foci was found in only 33% of trauma patients with MOFS (9). These observations have led to a current hypothesis that implicates the intestinal bacteria as the origin of MOFS in critically ill patients.

The GI tract is commonly regarded as an organ system involved solely with the digestion and absorption of nutrients. However, investigations have demonstrated that this system also regulates and processes metabolic substances circulating through the splanchnic vasculature and is a major component of host defenses. The GI mucosa normally is an efficient barrier that prevents migration of microorganisms and their by-products into the systemic circulation. The epithelial cells of the intestinal mucosa are in constant renewal and thus are markedly affected by the availability of nutrients, the hormonal environment, and intestinal blood flow.

The most important stimulus for mucosal cell proliferation is the presence of nutrients in the intestinal lumen (10). The transit of a meal through the GI tract increases epithelial desquamation and enhances mucosal cell proliferation. Bowel rest due to starvation or administration of parenteral nutrition leads to villous atrophy (11), a reduction in cellularity, and a reduction in intestinal disaccharidase activities (12). Indirect effects of nutrients on the GI tract are mediated by enterohormones, such as gastrin, peptide YY, and enteroglucagon, and by nonenteric hormones, such as growth hormone and epidermal growth factor (13).

Nutrients taken up by enterocytes for cellular metabolism may enter the intestine through the luminal side or the basolateral membrane via the mesenteric arteries. Enterocytes extract glutamine that is oxidized in preference to glucose, fatty acids, or ketone bodies in the small intestine (14). Glutamine becomes available to the small intestine from mucosal absorption or systematically as a result of muscle proteolysis.

Colonocytes use n-butyrate, a short-chain fatty acid (SCFA), in preference to glutamine, glucose, and ketone bodies (15). In contrast to glutamine, which is synthesized by the body, butyrate is not produced by mammalian tissues and is only available to the colonic mucosa as a result of bacterial fermentation in the colonic lumen. The SCFA, primarily butyrate but also acetate and propionate, are utilized for energy-consuming cellular processes in the colon, such as sodium absorption and cell proliferation and growth (16,17).

Within the anaerobic environment of the colon, the preferred substrates for bacterial fermentation are carbohydrates, which normally reach the cecum in the form of dietary fiber or undigested starch. Intraluminal fermentation of fiber polysaccharides follows a stoichimetric equation (18):

$$34.5\ C_6H_{12}O_6 \rightarrow 64\ SCFA + 23.75\ CH_4 + 34.23\ CO_2 + 10.5\ H_2O$$

The methane (CH_4) produced is further converted to H_2O and CO_2. The three principal SCFA (acetate, propionate, and n-butyrate) are produced in a constant ratio of 1:0.3:0.25. These three SCFA account for approximately 83% of all SCFA produced (19).

The bacterial flora use less than 10% of the energy available from the fiber fermentation for metabolic activities, and the remaining energy is transferred into SCFA, which can be either absorbed or excreted in the feces (18). Based on in vivo perfusion studies, it is estimated that the human colon is able to absorb up to 540 kCal/day in the form of SCFA (20).

In the absence of the physical stimulus of a meal and the lack of intestinal fuels (e.g., glutamine and n-butyrate), the small (21) and large bowel (22) atrophy. This atrophy not only affects absorptive cells but also mucus-secreting cells, gut-associated lymphoid tissue (GALT), and brush border enzymes. Whereas brush border enzymes and absorptive cells are essential for nutrient assimilation, mucus cells and the GALT are key components of the intestinal barrier. Bacteria, endotoxins, and other antigenic macromolecules are contained in the intestinal lumen by this barrier.

The number and types of bacteria also influence the efficiency of the intestinal barrier. The upper GI tract is essentially devoid of bacteria as a result of the bactericidal action of hydrochloric acid in the stomach and the intestinal motility that sweeps any surviving bacteria toward the colon. In the human colon bacteria exist in counts as high as 10^{11}. The homeostasis of these bacteria is closely controlled by the availability of energy substrates, the physicochemical conditions of the colonic lumen, and the interactions among microorganisms with the microbial environment (23).

The disruption of the intestinal barrier and alteration of the bacterial microflora allow greater translocation of bacteria and absorption of endotoxins from the gut lumen (24). Bacterial translocation is the process of bacterial migration or invasion across the intestinal mucosa into mesenteric lymph nodes and the portal bloodstream. Bacterial translocation has been studied most extensively in animal models. In a rat model of 40% scald burn, enteric bacteria were demonstrated in mesenteric lymph nodes and the spleen (25). Bowel rest with parenteral nutrition produced bacterial translocation in rats by increasing the cecal bacterial counts and impairing the intestinal barrier (26).

Bacteriologic cultures in portal blood obtained intraoperatively were positive in more than 30% of patients undergoing surgery for noninflammatory lesions of the GI tract (27). Life-threatening infections from gut-associated bacteria have been documented in patients with MOFS (2), in those with cancer who have had chemotherapy (28), and in those with major burns (29).

Bacterial endotoxins may also migrate across the gut mucosa. Endotoxins are a lipopolysaccharide component of the bacterial cell wall, which are normally absorbed in small quantities into the bloodstream and efficiently detoxified by hepatic Kupferr's cells (30). Temporary occlusion of the superior mesenteric artery is a well-recognized model of circulatory shock. During and after intestinal ischemia the portal blood contains a potent factor, or factors, capable of inducing hypotension and shock. One of these factors has been identified as endotoxins (31–33).

Translocated bacteria and endotoxins gaining access to the systemic circulation activate the coagulation system, complement cascade, macrophages, and neutrophils. These systems, in turn, release the aforementioned mediators that trigger the sequential or simultaneous inflammatory response in multiple organs, establishing the link between intestinal barrier failure and MOFS (Figure 3-1).

INDICATIONS FOR ENTERAL NUTRITION IN CRITICALLY ILL PATIENTS

General indications for EN in critically ill patients include the presence of malnutrition, insufficient volitional intake, and a GI tract that can be used safely and effectively. The American Society for Parenteral and Enteral Nutrition (A.S.P.E.N.) has listed a number of conditions that are grouped in categories of responsiveness to EN. In critically ill patients, the indications are not as clear as in stable hospitalized patients. The indications have therefore been modified as shown in Table 3-1.

As described previously, critical illnesses are associated with numerous GI

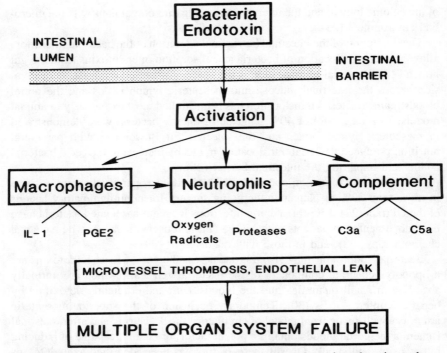

Figure 3-1. A schematic diagram of the linkage between bacteria endotoxins and multiple organ system failure (Reference 3, permission granted).

disorders in which EN may be beneficial in one patient and deleterious in another, despite both having the same GI disorder. For instance, stress gastritis, acalculous cholecystitis, ileus, and diarrhea are not absolute contraindications for EN. Furthermore, one could postulate that EN instituted early in the course of critical illnesses might help to prevent these complications. However, the decision to initiate EN in these patients is based upon a very thorough clinical and biochemical examination and other methods of diagnosis.

A patient with mild bleeding stress ulceration and hemodynamic stability can benefit from EN. Patients with ileus can be fed with EN as long as the diagnosis of mechanical obstruction has been eliminated and there is access to the small bowel for feeding with simultaneous gastric decompression.

Diarrhea in a critically ill patient is difficult when EN is considered for nutritional support. Diarrhea may be simply a consequence of prolonged bowel rest in which careful delivery of EN is warranted, but it also may indicate gut failure, with underlying ischemia and bacterial overgrowth, in which case EN is contraindicated.

TABLE 3-1. Indications for Enteral Nutrition in Critically Ill Patients

Hypermetabolism	Organ System Failure
Trauma	Respiratory (producing ventilator dependence)
Burn	Cardiac (resulting in cardiac cachexia)
Sepsis	Intestinal (caused by short bowel syndrome)
Postoperative major surgeries	Hepatic (resulting in hepatic encephalopathy)
Gastrointestinal Disease	Renal (producing uremia)
Esophageal obstruction	Central nervous system (resulting in coma)
Pancreatitis	
Inflammatory bowel disease	Multiple organ system failure
Fistulas	

From reference 3, with permission.

Most critical care specialists are now aware of the possibility of the gut being the origin of sepsis and MOFS. The suspicion arises when a patient develops enteric bacteremia and sepsis without discernible evidence of the source of sepsis. Such patients may be experiencing any phase of the MOFS with varying compromise of other organ systems. Based on clinical data (34), one can predict that a patient with isolated pulmonary failure is at an early stage of this syndrome, whereas a patient with renal failure and two or more organ failures is at the end stage of the spectrum.

The problem is compounded by the lack of confirmatory tests to aid in diagnoses of bacterial translocation and endotoxin transmigration. In deciding to provide EN, it may suffice to know whether or not there is underlying bacterial overgrowth of the small bowel. Breath hydrogen analysis is a simple, noninvasive test designed to assess bacterial overgrowth of the small bowel in a variety of chronic GI diseases. This test is being used in a few research centers to diagnose bacterial overgrowth in critically ill patients. The results of this test are confounded by motility disorders, and it is somewhat cumbersome in intubated patients. However, preliminary results with the breath hydrogen test are promising and it may become a useful measurement for the critically ill patient. Other methods being tested for assessing intestinal permeability include urinary excretion of lactulose and fecal clearance of $alpha_1$-antitrypsin.

If the patient is stable and fewer than two organ systems are affected, and bacterial overgrowth cannot be demonstrated, a trial of EN is warranted. These patients tolerate hyperosmolar and high-fat diets poorly; therefore, an isotonic (diluted) carbohydrate-based diet is initiated by continuous infusion at a rate of 20 ml/hr. The patient should be closely monitored not only for signs of diet intolerance but also for worsening of the MOFS. If the patient develops ileus, diarrhea worsens, or the organ failure syndrome continues to involve more systems, EN should be withheld. Intolerance to EN is associated with increased mortality in critically ill patients (35,36). Therefore, EN may be considered a "stress test" in critically ill patients. The development of symptoms of "gut failure" usually indicates a poor prognosis.

Regardless of the tolerance to EN, one should not plan to meet all nutritional requirements via the GI tract. Supplemental parenteral feeding is usually necessary to meet the patient's needs while concurrent delivery of EN provides progressive stimulation to the GI tract.

A prerequisite for initiating EN in critically ill patients is adequate cardiopulmonary stability. As mentioned previously, the provision of EN in patients in shock states may actually be harmful. For practical purposes we define cardiac stability as a cardiac index of more than 2 L/m^2, with a mean arterial blood pressure of more than 70 mmHg, without the need for alpha-sympathetic stimulation. Adequate pulmonary function is defined as arterial oxygen saturation of more than 95% on inspired concentrations of oxygen of less than 60% and with less than 5 cm of positive end-expiratory pressure (PEEP). These are some arbitrary criteria that, in our experience, indicate acceptable oxygen delivery to tissues.

Enteral nutrition is contraindicated if the patient has failure of more than two organ systems, with continuing sepsis unresponsive to therapy, and cardiopulmonary instability. In these patients it is unlikely that a hyperpermeable small bowel populated by bacteria would benefit from EN. Moreover, intraluminal nutrients may increase bacterial overgrowth and worsen the patient's condition. However, it is also unlikely that bowel rest would reduce bacterial translocation and endotoxin transmigration.

Nutritional intervention and management of the patient with intestinal barrier failure are controversial and the subject of research in many medical centers. Research groups are working on the provision of intestinal fuels such as glutamine (37), SCFA (38), and ketones (39) via the parenteral route. Hormones with trophic effects on the intestine are also being investigated (40).

The sequential response of the GI tract during critical illnesses and potential therapeutic interventions are shown in Figure 3-2. At the onset of most critical illnesses, the intestine "rests." The lack of intraluminal nutrients leads to mucosal atrophy and diminished digestion secretions. Stress and deficit of intestinal fuels are additional factors that lead to further atrophy of the gut mucosa. This initial phase of gut atrophy is reversed or ameliorated by the administration of early enteral feedings, as shown by a series of experiments performed in animal models of stress (41). Intestinal fuels added to enteral diets significantly reduce the

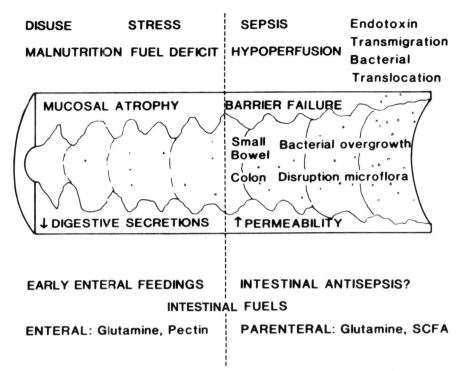

Figure 3-2. Schematic representation of the effects of critical illnesses on the gastrointestinal tract. On the upper part of the figure various noxious stimuli are listed in order of severity as the critical illness progresses. On the lower part of the figure potential therapeutic interventions are indicated during the progression of critical illness. The dotted vertical line represents an arbitrary point of irreversibility of the intestinal compromise, where the therapeutic approach changes from intraluminal nutrition to intestinal antisepsis and intravenous provision of intestinal fuels (Reference 3, permission granted).

atrophy due to lack of luminal nutrients and may further increase intestinal trophism.

As the critical illness progresses, the blood flow to the intestine is compromised, the lumen of the small intestine becomes colonized by bacteria, and the colonic microflora are disrupted. These derangements lead to increased permeability with translocation of bacteria and transmigration of endotoxins. This stage is known as "barrier failure." The vertical dotted line in Figure 3-2 represents an arbitrary point after which intraluminal manipulations not only may be ineffective but also may be deleterious.

SUMMARY

Nutritional support is a mandatory component in the care of critically ill patients. The gut is now known to be a potential source of sepsis in the critically ill patient, and this may be due to the disruption of the intestinal barrier. Because of the well-documented enterotrophic effects of intraluminal nutrients, evidence is accumulating to recommend the use of at least small amounts of enteral nutrition in selected patients with critical illnesses. However, critically ill patients often present with GI disturbances that preclude EN. A thorough understanding of the wide range of GI dysfunction during critical illness is required in order to prescribe enteral feeding safely and efficaciously. Before one initiates enteral feeding, the severity and reversibility of the critical condition should be evaluated.

REFERENCES

1. Cerra FB: Hypermetabolism, organ failure, and metabolic support. Surgery 101:1–14, 1987.
2. Marshall JC, Christou NV, Horn R, et al: The microbiology of multiple organ failure. Arch Surg 123:309–315, 1988.
3. Rolandelli RH, de Paula JA, Guenter P, Rombeau JL: Critical illness and sepsis, in Rombeau JL, Caldwell MD (eds) Clinical Nutrition: Enteral and Tube Feeding. Philadelphia: WB Saunders, 1990 pp. 288–305.
4. Gottlieb JE, Menashe PI, Cruze E: Gastrointestinal complications in critically ill patients: The intensivists' overview. Am J Gastroenterol 81:227–238, 1986.
5. Furness JB, Costa M: Adynamic ileus, its pathogenesis and treatment. Med Biol 52:82–89, 1974.
6. Smith J, Kelly KA, Weinshilboum RM: Pathophysiology of postoperative ileus. Arch Surg 112:203–209, 1977.
7. Vantrappen G, Janssens J, Hellemans J, et al: The interdigestive motor complex of normal subjects and patients with bacterial overgrowth of the small intestine. J Clin Invest 59:1158–1166, 1977.
8. Church JM, Fazio VW: The significance of quantitative results of *C. difficile* cultures and toxin assays in patients with diarrhea. Dis Colon Rectum 28:765–769, 1985.
9. Goris RJA, Boekholtz WKF, van Bebber IPT, et al: Multiple-organ failure and sepsis without bacteria. Arch Surg 121:897–901, 1986.
10. Johnson LR: Regulation of gastrointestinal mucosal growth. Physiol Rev 68:456–502, 1988.
11. Levine GM, Deren JJ, Steiger E, et al: Role of oral intake in maintenance of gut mass and disaccharidase activity. Gastroenterology 67:975–982, 1974.

12. Raul JA, Noriegar R, Doffeol M, et al: Modifications of brush border enzyme activities during starvation in the jejunum and ileum of adult rats. Enzyme 28:328–335, 1982.
13. Al-Nafussi AI, Wright NA: The effect of epidermal growth factor (EGF) on cell proliferation of the gastrointestinal mucosa of rodents. Virchows Arch B Cell Pathol 40:63–69, 1982.
14. Windmueller HG, Spaeth AE: Uptake and metabolism of plasma glutamine by the small intestine. J Biol Chem 249:5070–5079, 1974.
15. Roediger WEW: Utilization of nutrients by isolated epithelial cells of the rat colon. Gastroenterology 83:424–429, 1982.
16. Roediger WEW, Rae DA: Trophic effect of short-chain fatty acids on mucosal handling of ions by the defunctioned colon. Br J Surg 69:23–25, 1982.
17. Sakata T, Yajima T: Influence of short-chain fatty acids on the epithelial cell division of digestive tract. Br J Exp Physiol 69:639–648, 1984.
18. Miller, TL, Wolin MJ: Fermentation by saccharolytic intestinal bacteria. Am J Clin Nutr 32:164–172, 1979.
19. Cummings JH: Short-chain fatty acids in the human colon. Gut 763–779, 1981.
20. Ruppin H, Bar-Meir S, Soergel KH, et al: Absorption of short-chain fatty acids by the colon. Gastroenterology 78:11500–1507, 1980.
21. Ecknauer R, Sircar B, Johnson LR: Effect of dietary bulk on small intestinal morphology and cell renewal in the rat. Gastroenterology 81:781–786, 1981.
22. Ryan GP, Dudrick SJ, Copeland EM, et al: Effect of various diets on colonic growth in rats. Gastroenterology 77:458–463, 1979.
23. Savage DC: Gastrointestinal microflora in mammalian nutrition. Annu Rev Nutr 6:155–178, 1986.
24. Berg RD: Promotion of the translocation of enteric bacteria from the gastrointestinal tracts of mice by oral treatment with penicillin, clindamycin, or metronidazole. Infect Immun 33:854–861, 1981.
25. Maejima K, Deitch EA, and Berg RD: Bacterial translocation from the gastrointestinal tracts of rats receiving thermal injury. Infect Immun 43:6–10, 1984.
26. Alverdy JC, Aoys E, Moss GS: Total parenteral nutrition promotes bacterial translocation from the gut. Surgery 104:185–190, 1988.
27. Schatten WE, Desprez JD, Holden WD: A bacteriologic study of portal-vein blood in man. Arch Surg 71:404–409, 1955.
28. Bodey GP: Antibiotic prophylaxis in cancer patients: regimens of oral, nonabsorbable antibiotics for the prevention of infection during induction of remission. Rev Infect Dis 3 (suppl):S259, 1981.
29. Jarret F, Balish L, Moylan JA, et al: Clinical experience with prophylactic antibiotic bowel suppression in burn patients. Surgery 83:523, 1978.
30. Nolan JP: The contribution of gut-derived endotoxins to liver injury. Yale J Biol Med 52:106–112, 1985.

31. Lin MK, Zweifach WB: Results of pretreatment with antibiotics on survival following mesenteric arterial occlusion in rats. Proc Soc Exp Biol Med 108:27–31, 1976.
32. Cuevas P, de la Maza LM, Gilbert J et al: The lung lesion in four different types of shock in rabbits. Arch Surg 104:319–322, 1972.
33. Amudsen E, and Gustafsson B: Results of experimental intestinal strangulation obstruction in germ-free rats. J Exp Med 117:823–831, 1963.
34. Fry DE: Multiple system organ failure. Surg Clin North Am 68:107–122, 1988.
35. Chang RWS, Jacobs S, Lee B: Gastrointestinal dysfunction among intensive care unit patients. Crit Care Med 15:909–914, 1987.
36. Border JR, Hassett J, Laduca J, et al: The gut origin septic states in blunt multiple trauma (ISS=40) in the ICU. Ann Surg 206:427–448, 1987.
37. Hwang TL, O'Dwyer ST, Smith RJ et al: Preservation of small bowel mucosa using glutamine enriched parenteral nutrition. Surg Forum 37:56–58, 1986.
38. Koruda MJ, Rolandelli RH, Settle RG, et al: The effect of parenteral nutrition supplemented with short-chain fatty acids on adaptation to massive small bowel resection. Gastroenterology 95:710–720, 1988.
39. Kripke SA: Personal communication.
40. Wilmore DW, Smith RJ, O'Dwyer ST, et al: The gut: a central organ after surgical stress. Surgery 104:917–923, 1988.
41. Mochizuki H, Trocki O, Dominioni L, et al: Mechanism of prevention of postburn hypercatabolism by early enteral feeding. Ann Surg 200:297–310, 1984.

Requirements for Patients Receiving Enteral Nutrition

CHAPTER 4

Scott A. Shikora, M.D.

INTRODUCTION

Since the late 1960s, total parenteral nutrition (TPN) has been the gold standard for nutritional support. It can be administered safely and has become an integral part of the care of malnourished or critically ill hospitalized patients. Over the past decade, enterally administered nutritional support has gained considerable attention. Its favorable characteristics, such as its low complication rate, simplicity of delivery, and low cost, have been known for some time (1). Enteral nutrition has recently gained new popularity. Many publications describe the importance of maintaining gut mucosal integrity by the infusion of nutrients intraluminally for organism homeostasis and immunologic competence (2–5). In addition, the ability to utilize the GI tract in the immediate postoperative period has been shown to decrease metabolic rate (4,6,7) and improve nitrogen balance (3,8,9). In all probability, enterally administered nutrition will someday obtain at least an equal, and possibly, even a superior position to TPN in the care of hospitalized patients requiring nutritional support.

To be seriously considered as a primary nutritional modality, enteral nutrition must be able to satisfy the following three criteria:

1. It must be safe and its administration free of serious side effects.
2. It must be capable of fulfilling all macronutrient and micronutrient requirements.
3. It should be capable of being modified to meet special disease-specific limitations.

Accessible to the health care provider today are a multitude of commercially prepared enteral products. When practitioners have the proper knowledge of the nutritional requirements for hospitalized patients and the specific needs associated with certain disease states, these products can be used safely and successfully in most circumstances. The clinician interested in nutritional support must therefore have a thorough understanding of nutritional requirements.

Although most of the work to define calorie and nutrient needs was performed to address parenteral nutrition, there is no evidence to suggest that these recommendations cannot apply to enteral nutrition. The concerns regarding parenteral overfeeding are rarely an issue with enteral nutrition; however, the potential for complications associated with underfeeding is no less significant. Therefore, a careful prediction or actual measurement of caloric and substrate requirements is equally as important with either modality.

NUTRITIONAL ASSESSMENT

Nutritional support is not necessary for the majority of hospitalized patients. In most circumstances, a well-nourished patient in good health can withstand the effects of about 1 week of starvation and stress secondary to surgery, trauma, or illness (8). Nutritional intervention is indicated for the following subgroups of patients:

1. Patients found to be malnourished secondary to advanced age or comorbid disease states.
2. Patients who have had inadequate nutrition for greater than a week while in the hospital and do not seem capable of meeting nutritional requirements in the near future.
3. Patients who are critically ill and hypercatabolic.
4. Patients who, due to underlying disease states, will be at risk for long-term nutritional deficiencies.

Males: $REE = 66.5 + 13.8W + 5.0H - 6.8A$

Females: $REE = 655.1 + 9.6W + 1.8H - 4.7A$

Figure 4-1. The Harris-Benedict equation for estimating resting energy expenditure (REE). W=weight in kg, H=height in cm, and A=age in years. This formula was derived from measurements made in healthy volunteers.

The philosophy at our institution is to perform a comprehensive preoperative nutritional assessment on each patient considered for nutritional support. This includes a careful history with emphasis on significant weight loss (10% of usual body weight in the last 6 months), comorbidity, and a physical examination looking for signs of generalized muscle wasting. The appropriate laboratory studies drawn include the serum albumin, transferrin, and total lymphocyte counts. Other important variables such as the arm anthropometry, creatinine height index, and delayed hypersensitivity response to common skin antigens are also scrutinized (8,10).

CALORIC REQUIREMENTS

The original intent of parenteral nutrition was to provide nutrients substantially in excess of actual requirements. This was based on the assumption that patients requiring nutritional intervention were severely depleted and required aggressive repletion, thus the name "hyperalimentation." It has since been determined that such overfeeding was in fact dangerous and nutritional support should be titrated to match actual metabolic requirements (11). Many derived formulas have since been proposed to estimate caloric goals. One of the most widely used, the Harris-Benedict equation (12) predicts resting energy expenditure based on patient's age, gender, height, and weight (Figure 4-1). This formula was derived from work performed on 230 normal healthy postprandial subjects. Therefore, it does not account for the increased metabolic demand of stress or sepsis, nor does it consider the thermic effect of feeding. Several stress factors have subsequently been incorporated into the calculation to account for the influence of these variables, for example, multiplying the predicted caloric requirements by 1.2 for patients recovering from minor surgery, 1.6 for septic patients, and 2.1 for patients after major thermal burns. Although the addition of such factors has been shown in some studies to improve the accuracy for predicting caloric goals, other studies dispute this claim (13,14). Recent papers have also questioned the magnitude of the increase in the metabolic rate seen in stressed patients (15).

Another criticism of the Harris-Benedict equation and related formulas is the reliance on patients' height, weight, and/or body surface area. These factors can vary according to body fluid status, particularly in critically ill patients. An increase in body water will increase both body weight and surface area without increasing metabolically active tissue. This situation is seen with frequency in the critically ill patient. The use of these formulas in this setting can lead to the overestimation of metabolic rate (16). Shanbhogue et al. (17) described the use of 24-hr urinary creatinine excretion (which correlates well with lean body mass) in patients with normal renal function to estimate needs. This method seems to be better suited for critically ill malnourished patients.

Although numerous studies have examined the accuracy of many of the reported formulas to estimate metabolic rate, the consensus is that these formulas become increasingly inaccurate as the severity of illness increases (16). Therefore, although they can probably be used safely for most patients, in the critically ill, in whom the margin of safety is quite narrow, a more accurate modality is required.

The best method for determining caloric needs is the direct measurement of energy expenditure by indirect calorimetry (11,18). With the use of a portable gas analyzer or "metabolic cart," resting energy expenditure can easily be determined at the bedside. Since many facilities lack this technology, some accurate means of estimating needs remains necessary. Using actual measurements, it has been determined that the average-sized patient lying comfortably in bed requires about 23 kCal/kg body weight/day (8). This increases only slightly with most elective surgical procedures (11,19). The energy requirements of the most hypermetabolic (those patients with major sepsis or significant thermal burn) increases only to about 40–50 kCal/kg/day (8,10,19). Therefore, at many centers, including this institution, most patients are supplied 25–30 kCal/kg/day (10). This starting point can then be adjusted based on the patient's condition, or by actual measurements.

The need to meet caloric requirements cannot be overemphasized. Underfeeding will lead to continued weight loss, poor healing, sepsis, protein wasting, and, ultimately, organ failure and death. Overfeeding, although less of an issue with enteral nutrition, can still lead to troubling hyperglycemia, gastrointestinal intolerance, and volume overload. Whether nutrients are administered parenterally or enterally, the best nutritional goal remains the provision of the appropriate amount of calories required to meet energy demands and protein to reduce nitrogen losses.

MACRONUTRIENT REQUIREMENTS

Protein

Central to comprehensive nutritional intervention is the provision of protein. Dietary amino acids are mandatory as an energy fuel, in addition to being

$$\text{Nbal (g/d)} = \frac{\text{Protein Intake (g/d)}}{6.25} - [\text{UUN (g/d)} + \text{ANL (g/d)} + 4]$$

Figure 4-2. Formula for calculating nitrogen balance (Nbal). UUN=urine urea nitrogen. Abnormal nitrogen losses (ANL) include fistula output, wound exudates, dialysates, diarrhea or gastric losses.

irreplaceable for the maintenance of organ integrity, immunocompetence, and as the building blocks for wound healing (8,20). As with caloric requirements, the estimation of protein needs must be accurate. Insufficient administration can lead to persistent nitrogen wasting (18,21), the results of which are organ failure, sepsis, and subsequent death. The provision of excessive protein does not enhance uptake and may lead to increased ureagenesis, which can cause renal injury in some patients (18,21,22). Recent studies have supported the administration of approximately 1.5–2.0 g protein/kg body weight/day (8,10,21,23,24). Patients rarely require more. The ability to measure 24-hr urinary nitrogen excretion enables the clinician to adjust the amount on the basis of nitrogen losses (Figure 4-2). Total nitrogen excretion is the sum of the urine urea nitrogen, fecal, skin, and respiratory tract nitrogen losses (a factor of 2–4 grams), and any abnormal nitrogen losses such as fistula output, wound exudates, dialysates, diarrhea, or gastric tube losses (8). The goal is to match losses during the catabolic phase of illness, and to replete lost lean body mass during the anabolic phase. Achieving a "positive" nitrogen balance is virtually impossible in patients with continuing illness but is obtainable after the illness has resolved. Serial measurements can be performed, for example, weekly, and protein provision adjusted as indicated. This is particularly useful since patients might require various amounts of dietary nitrogen as their condition changes.

In certain subgroups of patients, such as those with renal or hepatic disease, protein administration might need to be kept intentionally below usual estimates. These patients have impaired nitrogen metabolism. The provision of protein in levels exceeding 0.8–1.0 g/kg/day can lead to worsening renal function or encephalopathy in patients with renal or hepatic disease, respectively.

Many of the currently available most popular commercial enteral feeds can only meet protein goals at high caloric and volume loads. Therefore, the potential to provide protein in significant excess of needs is difficult. In cases in which administration is inadequate, the addition of concentrated protein supplements such as Propac or Promed to the formulation will increase protein density without the burden of excessive calories or volume.

Also available are enteral products with unique protein formulations. Some contain high concentrations of branched chain amino acids, namely leucine, isoleucine, and valine. There is evidence that these amino acids increase protein synthesis and improve nitrogen balance at lower protein concentrations (23).

Some believe that their use is beneficial in patients with renal or hepatic disease (1). Glutamine, a key nonessential amino acid, has been shown to be the preferred respiratory fuel of the enterocyte (5). Formulations rich in glutamine, such as Vivonex, might offer some advantage over other feeds. In addition, arginine-enriched feedings may become popular since this amino acid is thought to modulate the immune system (25).

The complexity of the protein contained in the enteral product is also important. Most contain intact proteins (polymeric) that are well tolerated and absorbed by most patients. Certain patients, such as those with altered gastrointestinal function and those with intestinal mucosal atrophy secondary to prolonged disuse, might be intolerant to intact proteins. These patients would benefit from monomeric products such as Vivonex, which contains free amino acids, or Vital, which contains dipeptides and tripeptides of high biological value. These products are better tolerated since simple protein sources are readily absorbed without the need for complex digestion (6,8).

Carbohydrate

Glucose, the simplest form of carbohydrate, is the preferred fuel for many metabolically active organ systems including the central nervous system, the immune system, as well as the healing wound (11,20). In times of stress or injury, the importance of a readily available supply of glucose is magnified. When availability is deficient, the body will enhance its rate of gluconeogenesis to produce the needed amount of glucose. This results in increased protein catabolism and nitrogen wasting, with its inherent complications.

Although carbohydrates usually provide the majority of the calories administered, excessive carbohydrate provision is not without risks. This problem, although less common with the addition of fats to the nutritional admixtures, can still occur and must be avoided. The overconsumption of parenteral glucose has been shown to enhance lipogenesis, cause hepatic steatosis and subsequent hepatic dysfunction, exacerbate hyperglycemia in glucose-intolerant patients, and increase the production of CO_2 which can compromise respiration in patients with pulmonary disease (10,11,15,18,26,27).

The optimal amount of carbohydrate utilization has been determined. Wolfe et al. (28) have shown that patients do not oxidize more than 5–7 mg glucose/kg body weight/min given intravenously. Any rate of administration higher than this leads to storage. Initially, the excess is used to replete glycogen stores in the liver. Since this is a finite glucose pool, it is quickly replenished and the body then converts all excess glucose into triglyceride. Therefore, in most circumstances, the rate of infusion should not exceed about 4–5 mg/kg/min. In the average-sized patient, daily provision should be no greater than 300–400 g/day (10). Higher concentrations given enterally may exacerbate hyperglycemia in glucose-intolerant patients.

Dextrose is the glucose source in parenteral solutions; complex carbohydrates are used in most enteral feeds. They are usually well absorbed in the proximal small intestine. Some patients may exhibit intolerance to lactose, which can be seen after major small bowel resection, and is due to loss of the brush-border enzyme lactase (29,30).

Fat

With the addition of fat to both enteral and parenteral formulas, caloric goals can be achieved with less potential for carbohydrate overfeed. Thirty to 40% of caloric requirements is usually supplied by lipids. However, as with the other nutritional substrates, it must be used in a judicious manner. The provision of lipids, usually as long-chain triglycerides, has been associated with immunologic abnormalities including reticuloendothelial system dysfunction (14,31,32). This appears to be related to the amount and rapidity of administration. Lipids given intravenously over 24 hr continuously, and at concentrations less than 50% of the nonprotein calories, have been shown to be safe (15,31,33). This problem may not be as worrisome when the enteral route of nutritional support is chosen; however, long-chain triglycerides in enteral formulations maybe poorly tolerated in many patients secondary to the complex interplay between lipase, bile salts, and intestinal mucosa required for digestion and absorption. Patients with intestinal derangements such as postsurgical alterations, biliary or pancreatic disease, or intestinal mucosal diseases are the most susceptible (30). In addition, patients who develop mucosal atrophy following prolonged gastrointestinal disuse will have difficulty with formulas high in long-chain triglycerides. Intolerance usually presents as abdominal cramping, bloating, diarrhea, and steatorrhea. Long-chain triglycerides may also exacerbate gastroparesis in diabetic patients when infused directly into the stomach.

Other forms of lipid such as medium-chain triglycerides (MCT) are more easily absorbed (23,30,31). These require less absorption and do not influence reticuloendothelial function (15,31,33). Popular commercial products such as Vital contain high concentrations of MCT and are usually well tolerated in difficult-to-treat patients. We usually initiate enteral supplementation with a formula such as Vital, and then convert to a more conventional formula as tolerated. A patient on a long-term elemental formula can develop an essential fatty acid deficiency since MCT does not contain essential fatty acids.

In the future, one can expect to see enteral formulas containing fish oils and structured lipids, both of which have been shown to have beneficial effects (31).

MICRONUTRIENT REQUIREMENTS

Most commercially available enteral formulations provide the recommended daily allowance (RDA) of vitamins and trace elements. Therefore, they are sufficient without further supplementation for the majority of patients. Some patients, such as those with inappropriately high losses, (i.e., short bowel syndrome, high-output small intestinal fistula or ileostomies, malabsorption), as well as those with severe malnutrition, might require additional supplementation.

CONCLUSION

There are relatively few contraindications to administering nutritional support enterally. Gut utilization in the immediate postoperative period, long thought to be inappropriate, has been shown to be safe and even beneficial. Recent technologic advances include the new small-bore flexible catheters and portable infusion pumps have greatly simplified delivery. Many access options are available to meet specific patient requirements. These include nasal, percutaneous and operative placement for gastric or enteric catheters. All are easy to care for, safe, and amenable to home use.

Therefore, with the proper understanding of the basic nutritional requirements, and a knowledge of the various commercially available enteral formulations, few patients should be deprived of the benefits of enterally administered nutrients.

REFERENCES

1. Shanbhogue LKR, Bistrian BR, Blackburn GL: Trends in enteral nutrition in the surgical patient. J R Coll Surg Edinb 31:267, 1986.
2. Alverdy JC: The GI tract as an immunologic organ. Contemp Surg 35 (supp): 14, 1989.
3. Moore EE, Jones TN: Benefits of immediate jejunostomy feeding after major abdominal trauma-A prospective, randomized study. J Trauma 26:874, 1986.
4. Wilmore DW, Smith RJ, O'Dwyer ST, et al: The gut: a central organ after surgical stress. Surgery 104:917, 1988.
5. Souba WW: The gut—a key metabolic organ following surgical stress. Contemp Surg 35(suppl):5, 1989.
6. Blackburn GL, Bell SJ, Georgieff M: Enteral tube feeding: state of the art. Gastroenterology 23:7, 1985.
7. Glucksman DL, Kalser MH, Warren WD: Small intestinal absorption in the immediate postoperative period. Surgery 60:1020, 1966.
8. Blackburn GL: Nutrition in surgical patients, in Hardy JD, Kukora JS, Pass HI (eds) Hardy's Textbook of Surgery, ed 2. Philadelphia: JB Lippincott, 1988, p. 86.
9. Hoover HC, Ryan JA, Anderson EJ, et al: Nutritional benefits of immediate postoperative jejunal feeding of an elemental diet. Am J Surg 139:153, 1980.

10. Shanbhogue LKR, Chwals WJ, Weintraub M: Parenteral nutrition in the surgical patient. Br J Surg 74:172, 1987.
11. Hill GL, Church J: Energy and protein requirements of general surgical patients requiring intravenous nutrition. Br J Surg 71:1, 1984.
12. Harris JA, Benedict FG: Standard Basal Metabolism Constants for Physiologists and Clinicians, A Biometric Study of Basal Metabolism in Man. Philadelphia: JB Lippincott, 1919, p. 223.
13. Quebbeman EJ, Ausman RK, Schneider TC: A re-evaluation of energy expenditure during parenteral nutrition. Ann Surg 195:282, 1982.
14. Weissman C, Kemper M, Askanazi J, et al: Resting metabolic rate of the critically ill patient: Measured versus predicted. Anesthesiology 64:670, 1986.
15. McMahon MM, Benotti PN, Bistrian BR: A clinical application of exercise physiology and nutritional support for the mechanically ventilated patient. JPEN 14:538, 1990.
16. Damask MC, Schwarz Y, Weissman C: Energy measurements and requirements of critically ill patients, Crit Care Clin 3:71, 1987.
17. Shanbhogue LKR, Chwals WJ, Weintraub M, Blackburn GL, Blstrian BR: Parenteral nutrition in the surgical patient. Br J Surg 1987; 172–180.
18. Cerra FB: Hypermetabolism, organ failure, and metabolic support. Surgery 92:1, 1987.
19. Elwyn DH: Nutritional requirements of adult surgical patients. Crit Care Med 8:9, 1980.
20. Hensle TW, Askanazi J: Metabolism and nutrition in the perioperative period. J Urol 139:229, 1988.
21. Wolfe RR, Goodenough RD, Burke JF, et al: Response of protein and urea kinetics to different levels of protein intake. Ann Surg 197:163, 1983.
22. Shaw JHF, Wolfe RR: Whole-body protein kinetics in patients with early and advanced gastrointestinal cancer: The response to glucose infusion and total parenteral nutrition. Surgery 103:148, 1988.
23. Cerra FB, Upson D, Angelico R, et al: Branched chains support postoperative protein synthesis. Surgery 92:192, 1982.
24. Shizgal HM: Nutritional complications in the surgical patient, in Hardy JD (ed): Complications in Surgery and Their Management, ed 4. Philadelphia: WB Saunders, 1981, p. 245.
25. Daly JM, Reynolds J, Thom A, et al: Immune and metabolic effects of arginine in the surgical patient. Ann Surg 208:512, 1988.
26. Askanazi J, Rosenbaum SH, Hyman AI, et al: Respiratory changes induced by the large glucose loads of total parenteral nutrition. JAMA 243:1444, 1980.
27. Baker AL, Rosenberg IH: Hepatic complications of total parenteral nutrition. Am J Med 82:489, 1987.

28. Wolfe RR, O'Donnell TF, Stone MD, et al: Investigation of factors determining the optimal glucose infusion rate in total parenteral nutrition. Metabolism 29:892, 1980.
29. Weser E, Urban E: The short bowel syndrome, in Berk JE, Haubrich WS, Kalser MH, et al (eds): Bockus Gastroenterology, ed 4. Philadelphia: WB Saunders, 1985, p. 1792.
30. French AB, Cook HB, Pollard HM: Nutritional problems after gastrointestinal surgery. Med Clin North Am 53:1389, 1969.
31. Wan JM-F, Teo TC, Babayan VK, et al: Invited comment: lipids and the development of immune dysfunction and infection. JPEN 12(suppl):43s, 1988.
32. Alexander JW, Saito H, Trocki O, et al: The importance of lipid type in the diet after burn injury. Ann Surg 204:1, 1986.
33. Jensen GL, Mascioli EA, Seidner DL: Parenteral infusion of long- and medium-chain triglycerides and reticuloendothelial system function in man. JPEN 14:467, 1990.

Specific Nutrients for the Gastrointestinal Tract: Glutamine, Arginine, Nucleotides, and Structured Lipids

CHAPTER 5

Timothy J. Babineau, M.D.

INTRODUCTION

The concept of modifying dietary formulas to meet specific nutritional needs is not new. Efforts directed at disease prevention through diet manipulation date back through the history of Western civilization. Recent advances in our understanding of gastrointestinal (GI) physiology and immunology have led to the theory that patient-specific feeding with nutrient-specific formulas may offer immunologic and nutritional advantages over traditional "standard" enteral support. By modulating the enteral formulas patients receive, investigators are now seeking to augment the body's natural defense mechanisms to injury and illness. "Pharmacologic nutrition," based on our new understanding of the gut's role in critical illness, is gaining wide acceptance among clinicians dealing with malnourished, critically ill, hospitalized patients. In this chapter, we will review four specific nutrients purported to possess "pharmaconutritional" properties: arginine, glutamine, nucleotides, and structured lipids. Although a majority of the preliminary work has focused on the parenteral administration of these nutrients, newer information is becoming available on the role of these nutrients when administered via the gastrointestinal tract.

ARGININE

Pharmacologic actions of individual amino acids have recently received widespread attention. Arginine, in particular, has been the focus of intense research in both animals and humans regarding its role in immunoregulation and protein metabolism. Although not a traditional "essential" amino acid, it has been shown to be "semiessential" or "conditionally essential" under a variety of stress situations including burns, trauma, sepsis, and rapid growth (1,2).

Barbul and co-workers at Sinai Hospital have done much of the pioneering work to elucidate the role of this amino acid in both stressed and nonstressed states (3,4). On a biochemical level, arginine supports protein synthesis, biosynthesis of other amino acids, and, most importantly perhaps, urea formation. If not supplemented parenterally or enterally, arginine can be synthesized endogenously from ornithine via citrulline (5). Intestinal absorption of arginine, often in conjunction with lysine and ornithine, is energy- and sodium-dependent (6). Arginine levels within tissues are inversely related to arginase activity. The liver has high arginase activity and low arginine levels, while the kidney and muscles have low arginase activity but a relatively high arginine level (7). The reason for this difference is not known.

The exact daily nutritional requirements of arginine have not been clearly defined. Although dietary arginine is not essential for human survival and growth, certain clinical situations create a hormonal milieu in which arginine becomes conditionally essential for optimal growth, maintenance of protein metabolism, and positive nitrogen balance (8). A number of animal studies have documented arginine's role in growth and nitrogen retention in the starved or stressed state (9,10). Daly and co-workers have recently demonstrated similar effects in surgical patients (11). In addition to optimizing nitrogen balance, arginine is also known to have a protective effect against ammonia intoxication in rats (12). Arginine has multiple and potent secretagogue activities, including the increase of human pituitary growth hormone secretion, increased insulin release, increased glucagon release, and increased somatostatin release (13–15). Many of these activities are seen with intravenous administration of arginine only.

The majority of research involving arginine has focused on its ability to modulate the immune system of the stressed organism. In vitro studies have long shown that arginine is essential for the growth of cells in tissue culture (16). Work has recently focused on the relationship of dietary arginine supplementation to the immune status of animals and humans. The most profound effect of dietary arginine supplementation in animal studies has been its ability to increase thymic weight (through an increase in T lymphocytes) and thymocyte immune response (17–20). Reynolds and co-workers demonstrated that arginine-supplemented diets enhanced cytotoxic T lymphocyte development and increased Poly IC-inducible natural killer activity and kinetics of interleukin-2 (IL-2) receptor expression on activated T cells (21). Saito et al. showed that a diet supplemented with 2% arginine as total nonprotein calories resulted in increased survival, improved delayed hypersensitivity response, and improved local bacterial containment of subdermal staphylococcal injections in burned rats (22).

Studies have recently focused on the role of arginine-supplemented diets in humans. In 1981, Barbul and co-workers demonstrated that arginine-supplemented oral diets increased mean peripheral blood lymphocyte and blastogenic response to Concanavalin A (Con A) and Phytohemagglutinin (PHA) in 21 normal healthy human volunteers (23). Daly and co-workers in 1988 showed that 25 g arginine fed via a jejunal tube postoperatively to patients with cancer following major surgery resulted in positive nitrogen balance and increased lymphocyte response (increased CD4 cells and percentage of lymphocytes) (24). Alexander and co-workers found, in a prospective clinical study, that a diet with 2% arginine (as well as omega 3 fish oils) given to burned patients reduced wound infections, shorted hospital stay, and reduced death rates compared to standard enteral formulations (25,26). Whether this benefit was related to the 2% arginine or the omega 3 fish oil has not been clearly determined.

Arginine's role as both a nutrient and pharmacologic immune mediator is beginning to unfold. Further investigation is needed to determine dosage/response relationships and the bioavailability of arginine in both parenteral and enteral nutritional formulas. Most currently available enteral formulas (with the exception of IMPACT) contain only modest amounts of arginine. Until further studies have been completed, however, injudicious supplementation of arginine to standard enteral formulas is probably not warranted.

GLUTAMINE

Glutamine, a nonessential amino acid, is the most abundant amino acid in the body. Although nearly all tissues have the ability to synthesize glutamine de novo, certain disease states are associated with increased uptake of glutamine by cells. Studies in a variety of animals show that the gut's uptake of glutamine, particularly in the stressed state, far exceeds that of any other amino acid and that glutamine is the main respiratory fuel for the gut (27). This increased uptake, particularly in the enterocyte, is believed to play a role in the support of cellular metabolism and function (28). Recent work has demonstrated that glutamine may be beneficial, if not required, during certain critical illnesses (29,30). This has led to a reclassification of glutamine, which, like arginine, is now being considered a "conditionally essential" amino acid.

Glutamine serves multiple functions including nitrogen exchange between tissues, regulation of protein synthesis, and provision of a precursor in nucleotide synthesis (31–33). In addition, its role as a preferred fuel source for the enterocyte has been well documented (34,35). Numerous studies are being conducted to evaluate the effects of glutamine-enriched enteral and parenteral formulas in different clinical situations.

The metabolic processes of hypermetabolism have become increasingly categorized and understood. The realization that currently available total parenteral nutrition (TPN) solutions create a state of "bowel starvation" rather than "bowel rest" has led Dr. Souba at the University of Florida and Dr. Cerra at the University of Minnesota to popularize the central role of the gut in the metabolic response to injury (36–38). In the unstressed, well-nourished organism, the intestinal tract is able to maintain a barrier of entry to the microorganisms and toxins that reside within it. Critical illness, however, creates a hormonal and cytokine milieu that leads to gut mucosal atrophy, predisposing to bacterial escape from the bowel lumen and making the gut a potential source of infection (39). This concept of bacterial translocation in critical illness and its role in the initiation and propagation of multisystem organ failure (MSOF) has gained wide support (40,41). Glutamine's potential role in these events has been outlined by Souba, who has demonstrated that an "interorgan" glutamine cycle aimed at mobilizing glutamine stores during times of stress may exist. This cycle, if it exists, would serve to provide the glutamine necessary to aid in the repair of the injured gut mucosa and prevent further bacterial translocation. In addition, glutamine has been shown to play a role in the gut's lymphocyte proliferation, which characterizes the stress response.

A number of studies have documented that glutamine-enriched TPN formulas are safe and may help to maintain intestinal metabolism, structure, and function (42). Work has recently focused on glutamine-supplemented enteral formulas. The advantages of nutritional support via the enteral route over the parenteral route have been well documented (43,44), and attempts are being made to correlate the advantages of parenterally supplied glutamine with enterally supplied glutamine. However, unlike with parenterally supplied glutamine, animal studies have been largely unable to confirm the beneficial effects of glutamine-enriched enteral formulas on intestinal mucosal integrity and cell-mediated immune response. This may be because the benefits of enteral feeding per se outweigh any potential gain from glutamine alone. Van Buren and co-workers were unable to demonstrate a beneficial effect of enterally supplied glutamine on in vivo cell-mediated immune response (45). Cerra and co-workers could likewise find no difference in intestinal histologic appearance or the incidence of bacterial translocation in rats fed glutamine-enriched enteral formulas compared with those fed standard chow (glutamine content unknown) (46). Fox and co-workers did, however, show that a glutamine-supplemented enteral elemental diet prolonged survival of rats with experimentally induced enterocolitis and improved their nitrogen balance (47,48). Despite the conflicting data, good evidence exists that glutamine is a conditionally essential nutrient during times of stress. Further investigation is warranted to delineate its place in enteral formulas. At present however, glutamine's role in nutrition support centers around its ability to prevent gut mucosal atrophy in patents maintained solely on parenteral (glutamine-enriched) nutrition.

NUCLEOTIDES

Nucleotides, as the precursors of deoxyribonucleic acid (DNA) and ribonucleic acid (RNA), are the building blocks of life. Consisting of a nitrogen base, a sugar molecule, and one or more phosphate groups, nucleotides serve a multitude of important functions in cellular energetics and metabolism. Adenosine triphosphate (ATP), the major substance used by organisms for the transfer of chemical energy, is an adenine nucleotide. Until recently, nucleic acids (as sources of preformed purines and pyrimidines) were not considered essential for normal growth and development. Although the body is capable of de novo synthesis of purine and pyrimidine bases, animal studies have shown that a dietary requirement of preformed purine or pyrimidine bases may be required for normal development (49).

The metabolic fate of dietary purines and pyrimidines is currently being studied. The daily requirement for both purines and pyrimidines (from both biosynthesis and dietary) is estimated to be 450–700 mg/day in adults (50,51). A great deal more is known about the fate of dietary purines than pyrimidines due to the clinically toxic effects of purine's end catabolite, uric acid. Uric acid production parallels the amount of ingested purine. Pyrimidine's catabolites (B-alanine and B-aminoisobutyric acid), on the other hand, are either further catabolized or excreted, making them difficult to study. Both purines and pyrimidines have been shown to decrease de novo synthesis of these compounds in humans and animals when supplied enterally (52,53). Most currently available enteral formulas do not contain nucleotides, except those made from blended foods (i.e., meats, milks, etc.). Whether this has implications for the critically ill patient maintained solely by tube feeding is currently under investigation.

The role of dietary nucleotides in immune function, specifically lymphocyte metabolism, has been the focus of intense research. Van Buren and co-workers have demonstrated that dietary nucleotides were able to reverse malnutrition- and starvation-induced immunosuppression in rats (54). Van Buren's group also showed that helper/inducer T lymphocytes require exogenous nucleotides to respond normally following immune stimulation (55). In another study, Kulkarni et al. demonstrated that dietary nucleotide restriction negatively influenced the response of phagocytic cells to bacterial sepsis in mice (56). This relationship between nucleotide metabolism and lymphocytic activity has important clinical consequences currently being investigated in humans. Van Buren observed that patients who have received renal allografts and are supported with hyperalimentation (containing no nucleotide sources) displayed a suppressed immune response to the allograft even when traditional pharmacologic immunosuppression had been reduced (57). This observation was further documented in animal studies involving allograft survival and nucleotide-enriched (or depleted) formulas (58,59).

Dietary sources of nucleotides appear to be important to support optimal growth and function of metabolically active cells such as lymphocytes, macrophages, and intestinal cells. Nucleotide-free diets have been shown to improve survival after allograft transplantation, while nucleotide-rich diets have led to enhanced immune responses in mice. Further studies in humans are warranted to delineate the clinical usefulness of these observations.

STRUCTURED LIPIDS

Unlike protein and glucose metabolism, fat metabolism (particularly in critical illness) is just now beginning to be understood and, as Weiner et al. pointed out, "many of our observations can be described but not necessarily explained" (60). During critical illness, and in the absence of supplemented nutrition, the major source of energy is body fat. During the first 24 hrs after acute trauma, there is an increase in fat mobilization (lipolysis), serum free fatty acids (FFA), and fat oxidation (61). If the stress persists, a complex balance of increased lipolysis, increased lipogenesis from re-esterification, and substrate cycling ensues. Although fat metabolism is incompletely understood, problems resulting from overfeeding with dextrose-alone formulas had prompted the use of fats as a nonglucose energy source to create a mixed fuel system.

Lipids are an essential component of our body. Conventional fats and oils are composed of glycerides of long-chain fatty acids and are designated as long-chain triglycerides (LCTs). Enterally supplied long-chain triglycerides are hydrolyzed into long-chain fatty acids in the small intestine. These fatty acids then become re-esterified (in the intestinal cells) into triglycerides, which eventually reform into chylomicrons. These chylomicrons, acting as the transport vehicles for the LCTs, are deposited into the lymphatic system and gain access to the hepatic circulation via the hepatic artery. Polyunsaturated fatty acids with 16 and 18 carbons (i.e., soybean and safflower oil) are rich in omega 6 fatty acids. Most enteral formulas contain a 50:50 mix of LCTs and medium-chain triglycerides (MCTs), which will be discussed later. In contrast, intravenous TPN solutions contain lipid emulsions that are 100% LCTs. Such "conventional" lipids (particularly when given parenterally) have recently been incriminated as causing a number of untoward side effects in critically ill patients, thus prompting a search for "alternative" lipid sources.

Linoleic acid, a long-chain essential fatty acid, is found in most conventional lipid emulsion formulas. Through its conversion into arachidonic acid, linoleic acid serves as a precursor to prostanoids (particularly PGE2), thromboxanes of the 2 series, and leukotrienes of the 4 series. These compounds, largely proinflammatory, have been implicated as mediators in the vascular component of septic shock (62). Attempts to reduce, in particular, thromboxane 2 production, have led to investigations in altering eicosanoid metabolism, specifically through the provision of lipids containing the omega 3 fatty acids found principally in fish oils. Both the 20-carbon (omega 3) eicosapentaenoic acid and the 22-carbon (omega 3) compete with arachidonic acid for cyclo-oxygenase and lipoxygenase, yielding instead a 3 series of prostanoids and 5 series of leukotrienes. These latter compounds are much less inflammatory and vasoactive. For example, thromboxane A2 produced in platelets is a potent platelet aggregator and vasoconstrictor. Thromboxane A3, an end product of omega 3 fatty acid metabolism, is a moderate vasoconstrictor and does not aggregate platelets (63–65). More specifically, Endres has shown that fish oil supplementation of a normal diet in healthy volunteers could reduce the physiological effects of endotoxin as well as reduce the interleukin-1 and tumor necrosis factor production due to endotoxin stimulation in monocytes studied in vitro (66).

The ability of fish oil to modify the response to endotoxin has been further pioneered by Bistrian and co-workers, who have demonstrated that long-term oral feeding and short-term parenteral feeding of fish oil (compared to safflower oil) could improve survival in guinea pigs after a lethal dose of intraperitoneal endotoxin (67,68). Diets enriched with fish oil also ameliorated lactic acidosis following sublethal doses of endotoxin in guinea pigs (69). Parenteral feeding with fish oil was more effective in rapidly changing membrane composition in various tissues, presumably reflecting the persistent serum availability of fish oil's distinctive fatty acids (70). Studies are currently being conducted to evaluate these hypotheses in humans. One such study comparing two enteral diets (one containing fish oil [71]) has been presented in preliminary form and has demonstrated an improved clinical outcome in terms of infection and length of stay.

In addition to fish oil, structured lipids containing a balance of medium-chain and long-chain triglycerides are being developed. Medium chain triglycerides consist essentially of the 8-carbon fatty acid octanoic acid and the 10-carbon fatty acid decanoic acid. Medium-chain triglycerides are hydrolyzed in the small intestine into medium-chain fatty acids. These fatty acids then bind to serum albumin, enter the portal vein, and are transported directly to the liver where they are oxidized. In addition, medium-chain fatty acids are rapidly cleared from the blood, rapidly oxidized independent of carnitine transport, and poorly stored in adipose tissue (72–74). Re-esterified mixtures of MCT and LCT are used to form so-called "structured lipids." Work in animals has shown that parenterally administered structured lipids containing MCTs result in less reticuloendothelial system (RES) impairment, a lowered incidence of bacteremia, and an enhanced nitrogen-sparing response to stress (75,76). Studies in humans (using a physical mix of MCTs rather than structured lipids) have also documented that parenterally administered LCTs result in significant RES dysfunction compared with MCT solutions (77). Mascioli and co-workers have shown that TPN consisting of MCTs resulted in increased thermogenesis reflective of MCTs property as an obligate fuel (78).

The effects of enterally provided MCTs are only beginning to be examined. Initial data from animals have shown that enterally administered MCTs resulted in greater cumulative nitrogen balance in burned rats (79). In addition, Teo and co-workers demonstrated a lower overall metabolic rate when burned rats were fed a formula containing structured lipids composed of MCTs and fish oil (80). In a recent study, critically ill patients who were enterally fed a formula containing MCTs demonstrated a change in red blood cell phospholipid fatty acids when compared with a group that did not receive MCTs (81). Newer enteral products contain a variety of physical mixtures, each of which has a variety of metabolic implications. Prospective, randomized testing is currently being conducted to evaluate the efficacy of these different formulas.

CONCLUSION

It is clear from the dramatic discoveries over the past several years regarding GI mucosal integrity, immunotherapy, and modulated feedings that nutrition support no longer simply involves providing adequate protein and calories. Through dietary manipulations and "pharmaconutrition," investigators are working on modifying the body's response to stress and enhancing natural defense mechanisms. Discussed above are four specific nutrients (arginine, glutamine, nucleotides and structured lipids) that have been the focus of recent research. Randomized, prospective trials, which are currently being conducted, will elucidate the precise role, if any, these nutrients play in critical illness.

REFERENCES

1. Rose WC: The nutritive significance of the amino acids and certain related compounds. Science 86:298–300, 1937.

2. Rose WC: Amino acid requirements of man. Fed Proc 8:546–552, 1949.
3. Barbul A. Arginine: biochemistry, physiology, and therapeutic implications. JPEN 10:227–238, 1986.
4. Seifter E, Rettura G, Barbul A, et al. Arginine: an essential amino acid for injured rats. Surgery 84:224, 1978.
5. Ratner S: Enzymes of arginine and urea synthesis. Adv Enzymol 39:1–90, 1973.
6. Milne MD, Asatoor AM, Edwards KDG, et al: The intestinal absorption defect in cystinuria. Gut 2:323–337, 1961.
7. Gopalakrishna R, Nagarajan B: Effect of growth and differentiation on distribution or arginase and arginine in rat tissues. Indian J Biochem Biophys 16:66–68, 1979.
8. Nakagawa I, Takahashi T, Suzuki T, et al: Amino acid requirements of children: minimal needs of tryptophan, arginine and histidine based on nitrogen balance method. J Nutr 80:305, 1963.
9. Saito H, Trocki O, Wang S, et al: Metabolic and immune effects of dietary arginine supplementation after burn. Arch Surg 122:784–789, 1987.
10. Barbul A, Wasserkrug HL, Seifter E et al: Immunostimulatory effects of arginine in normal and injured rats. J Surg Res 29:228–235, 1980.
11. Daly JM, Reynolds J, Thom A et al: Immune and Metabolic Effects of Arginine in the Surgical Patient. Ann Surg 208:512–523, 1988.
12. du Ruisseaj JP, Greenstein JP, Winitz ME, et al: Studies on the metabolism of amino acids and related compounds in vivo. VI. Free amino acid levels in the tissues of rats protected against ammonia toxicity. Arch Biochem Biophys 68:161–171, 1957.
13. Merimee TJ, Rabinowitz D, Riggs L: Plasma growth hormone after arginine infusion: clinical experiences. N Engl J Med 267:434, 1967.
14. Palmer JP, Walter RM, Ensinck JW: Arginine-stimulated acute phase of insulin and glucagon secretion. I. In normal man. Diabetes 24:735, 1975.
15. Weir CB, Samols E, Loo S, et al: Somatostatin and pancreatic polypeptide secretion: effects of glucagon, insulin and arginine. Diabetes 28:35, 1979.
16. Eagle H: Amino acid metabolism in mammalian cell culture. Science 130:432, 1959.
17. Barbul A, Rettura G, Levenson SM, et al: Arginine: thymotropic and wound healing promoting agent. Surg Forum 28:101, 1977.
18. Barbul A, Wasserkrug HL, Sisto DA, et al: Thymic and immune stimulatory actions of arginine. JPEN 4:446, 1980.
19. Barbul A, Wasserkrug HL, Yoshimura NN, et al: High arginine levels in intravenous hyperalimentation abrogate post-traumatic immune suppression. J Surg Res 36:620, 1984.
20. Barbul A, Fishel RS, Shimazu S, et al: Intravenous hyperalimentation with high arginine levels improves wound healing and immune function. J Surg Res 31:328, 1985.

21. Reynolds JV, Zhang SM, Thom AK, et al: Arginine as an immunomodulator. Surg Forum 38:415, 1988.
22. Saito H, Trocki O, Wang S, et al: Metabolic and immune effects of dietary arginine supplementation after burn. Arch Surg 122:784, 1987.
23. Barbul A, Sisto DA, Wasserkrug HL: Arginine stimulates lymphocyte immune response in healthy humans. Surgery 90:244, 1981.
24. Daly JM, Reynolds J, Thoma A et al: Immune and metabolic effects of arginine in the surgical patient. Ann Surg 208:512–523, 1988.
25. Alexander JW, Gottschlich MM: Nutritional immunomodulation in burn patients. Crit Care Med 18:S149–S153, 1990.
26. Gottschlich MM, Jenkins M, Warden GD et al: Differential effects of three enteral dietary regiments on selected outcome variables in burn patients. JPEN 14:225–236, 1990.
27. Windmueller HG: Glutamine utilization by the small intestine. Adv Enzymol 53:201–237, 1982.
28. Bergstrom A, Furst P, Noree Lo, et al: Intracellular free amino acid concentration in human muscle tissue. J Appl Physiol 36:693, 1974.
29. Souba WW, Klimberg VS, Hautamaki RD, et al: Oral glutamine reduces bacterial translocation following abdominal radiation. J Surg Res 48:1–5, 1990.
30. Souba WW, Klimberg VS, Plumley DA, et al: The role of glutamine in maintaining gut structure and function and supporting the metabolic response to injury and infection. J Surg Res 48:383–391, 1990.
31. Souba WW: Interorgan ammonia metabolism in health and disease: a surgeon's view. JPEN 11:569, 1987.
32. Rennie MJ, MacLennan PA, Hundal HS, et al: Skeletal muscle glutamine transport, intramuscular glutamine concentration, and muscle protein turnover. Metabolism 38:47–51, 1989.
33. Martin DW: Metabolism of purine and pyrimidine nucleotides, in DW Martin et al (eds) Harper's Review of Biochemistry. New York: Lange Book Series, 1989, pp 331–348.
34. Souba WW, Scott TE, Wilmore DW: Intestinal consumption of intravenously administered fuels. JPEN 9:18–22, 1985.
35. Souba WW, Smith RJ, Wilmore DW: Glutamine metabolism by the intestinal tract. JPEN 9:608–17, 1985.
36. Souba WW, Herskowitz K, Austgen TR, et al. Glutamine nutrition: theoretical considerations and therapeutic impact. JPEN Suppl 14:237S–243S, 1990.
37. Cerra FB, Holman RT, Bankey PE et al., Nutritional pharmacology: its role in the hypermetabolism-organ failure syndrome. Crit Care Med 18:S154–S158, 1990.
38. Cerra FB: Hypermetabolism, organ failure, and metabolic support. Surgery 101:1–14, 1987.
39. Deitch EA, Winterton J, Li M, et al: The gut as a portal of entry for bacteremia: role of protein malnutrition. Ann Surg 205:681–692, 1987.

40. Alverdy JC, Aoys E, Moss GS: Effect of commercially available chemically defined liquid diets on the intestinal microflora and bacterial translocation from the gut. JPEN 14:1–5, 1990.
41. Alverdy JC, Aoys E, Moss G; Total parenteral nutrition promotes bacterial translocation from the gut. Surgery 104:185–90, 1988.
42. Lowe DK, Benfell K, Smith RJ, et al: Safety of glutamine-enriched parenteral nutrient solutions in humans. Am J Clin Nutr 52:1101–1106, 1990.
43. Saito H, Trocki O, Alexander JW: The effect of route of nutrient administration on the nutritional state, catabolic hormone secretion and gut mucosal integrity after burn injury. JPEN 11:1–7, 1987.
44. Borlase BC, Babineau TJ, Forse RA, et al: Enteral nutrition in the critically ill, in Rippe et al (eds) Intensive Care Medicine. Boston: Little, Brown, 1991.
45. Kulkarni AD, Kumar S, Pizzini RP, et al: Influence of dietary glutamine and IMPACT on in vivo cell-mediated immune response in mice. Symp Proc Suppl Nutr.
46. Wells CL, Jechorek RP, Erlandsen SL, et al: The effect of dietary glutamine and dietary RNA on ileal flora, ileal histology, and bacterial translocation in mice. Symp Proc. Suppl Nutr. 70–75.
47. Fox AD, Kripke SA, Berman JR, et al: Reduction of the severity of enterocolitis by glutamine-supplemented enteral diets. Surg Forum 38:43–44, 1987.
48. Fox AD, Kripke SA, DePaula J, et al: Effect of a glutamine-supplemented enteral diet on methotrexate-induced enterocolitis. JPEN 12:325–331, 1988.
49. Savaiano DA, Ho CY, Chu V, et al: Metabolism of orally and intravenously administered purines in rats. J. Nutr 110:1793, 1980.
50. Smith LH Jr: Pyrimidine metabolism in man. N Engl J Med 288:764, 1973.
51. Bono VH Jr, Weissman SM, Frei E III: The effect of 6-azauridine administration on de novo pyrimidine production in chronic myelogenous leukemia. J Clin Invest 43:1486, 1964.
52. Zollner N, Grobner W: Purine and Pyrimidine Metabolism. Amsterdam: Elsevier, 1977, p. 165.
53. Leleiko NS, Martin BA, Walsh M, et al: Tissue-specific gene expression results from a purine- and pyrimidine free diet and 6-mercaptopurine in the rat small intestine and colon. Gastroenterology 93:1014, 1987.
54. Pizzine RP, Kumar S, Kulkarni A, et al: Dietary nucleotides reverse malnutrition and starvation induced immunosuppression. Arch Surg 125:86–90, 1990.
55. Van Buren CT, Kulkarni AD, Fanslow WC, et al: Dietary nucleotides, a requirement for helper/inducer T lymphocytes. Transplantation 40:694–698, 1985.
56. Kulkarni AD, Fanslow WC, Drath DB, et al: Influence of dietary nucleotide restriction on bacterial sepsis and phagocytic cell function in mice. Arch Surg 121:169–172, 1986.
57. Van Buren CT, Kulkarni AD, Rudolph F: Synergistic effect of a nucleotide-free diet and cyclosporine on allograft survival. Transplant Proc Suppl 1–2:2967, 1983.

58. Van Buren CT, Kulkarni AD, Schandlle VP, et al: The influence of dietary nucleotides on cell-mediated immunity. Transplantation 36:350, 1983.
59. Van Buren CT, Kim E, Kulkarni AD, et al: Nucleotide-free diet and suppression of immune response. Transplant Proc Suppl 5:57, 1987.
60. Weiner M, Rothkopf MM, Rothkopf G, et al: Fat metabolism in injury and stress. Crit Care Clin 3:1–25, 1987.
61. Babineau TJ, Borlase BC, Blackburn GL: Applied total parenteral nutrition in the critically ill, in Rippe et al (eds) Intensive Care Medicine. Boston: Little, Brown, 1991.
62. Mertin J, Stackpoole A, Shumway S: Nutrition and immunity: the immuno-regulatory effect of n-6 essential fatty acids is mediated through prostaglandin E. Int Arch Allergy Appl Immunol 77:390–395, 1975.
63. Hanburg M, Svensson J, Wakabayshi T, et al: Isolation of and structure of two prostagglandin endoperoxides that cause aggregation. Proc Natl Acad Sci USA 71:345, 1979.
64. Fisher S, Weber PC: Thromboxane A3 is formed in human platelets after dietary eicosapentaenoic acid. Biochem Biophys Res Commun 116:1091, 1983.
65. Needleman P, Raz A, Minkes MS, et al: Triene prostaglandins: prostacyclin and thromboxane biosynthesis and unique biological properties. Proc Natl Acad Sci USA 76:944, 1979.
66. Endres S, Ghorbani R, Kelley VE, et al: Dietary N-3 polyunsaturated fatty acids suppress synthesis of interleukin-1 and tumor necrosis factor. N Engl J Med 320:265, 1989.
67. Mascioli EA, Iwasa Y, Trimbo S, et al: Effect of menhaden oil diet on survival to endotoxin in guinea pigs. Am J Clin Nutr 49:277, 1989.
68. Mascioli EA, Leader L, Flores E, et al: Enhanced survival to endotoxin in guinea pigs fed IV fish oil. Lipids 23:623, 1988.
69. Pomposelli JJ, Flores EA, Blackburn GL, et al: Diets enriched with N-3 fatty acids ameliorated lactic acidosis by improving endotoxin-induced tissue hypoperfusion in guinea pigs. Ann Surg 213:166, 1991.
70. Ling PR, Istfan NW, Lopes SM, et al: Structured lipid made from fish oil and medium chain triglycerides alters tumor and host metabolism in Yoshida-sarcoma-bearing rats. Am J Clin Nutr 53:1177, 1991.
71. Daly JM, Lieberman M, Golfine MS, et al: Enteral nutrition with supplemental arginine, RNA and omega-3 fatty acids: a prospective clinical trial (abstr). JPEN 15:17, 1991.
72. Mascioli EA, Bistrian BR, Babayan VK et al: Medium chain triglycerides and structured lipids as unique nonglucose energy sources in hyperalimentation. Lipids 22:421–23, 1987.
73. Bach AC, Babayan VK: Medium chain triglycerides: an update. Am J Clin Nutr. 36:950, 1982.

74. Bell SJ, Mascioli EA, Bistrian BR, et al: Alternative lipid sources for enteral and parenteral nutrition: Long and medium chain triglycerides, structured triglycerides and fish oils. J Am Dietet Assoc 91:1–74, 1991.
75. Hamawy KH, Moldawer LL, Georgieff M, et al: The effect of lipid emulsions on reticuloendothelial system function in the injured animal. JPEN 9:559–565, 1985.
76. Mok KT, Maiz A, Yamazaki K, et al: Structured medium-chain and long-chain triglyceride emulsions are superior to physical mixtures in sparing body protein in the burned rat. Metabolism 33:910–915, 1984.
77. Jensen GL, Mascioli EA, Seidner DL: Parenteral infusion of long- and medium-chain triglycerides and reticuloendothelial system function in man. JPEN 14:467–471, 1990.
78. Mascioli EA, Randall S, Porter K, et al: Thermogenesis from intravenous medium-chain triglycerides. JPEN 15:27–31, 1991.
79. DeMichele SJ, Karlstad MD, Babayan VK, et al: Enhanced skeletal muscle and liver protein synthesis with structure lipid in enterally fed burned rats. Metabolism 37:787–795, 1988.
80. Teo T, DeMichele S, Selleck K, et al: Administration of structured lipid (SL) composed of MCT and fish oil reduces net protein catabolism in interally fed burned rats. Ann Surg 210:100–107, 1989.
81. Diboune M, Ferard G, Ingenbleek Y, et al: Composition of phospholipid fatty acids in red blood cell membranes of patients in intensive care units: effects of different intakes of soybean oil, medium-chain triglycerides and black-currant seed oil. JPEN 16:136–141, 1992.

CLINICAL RATIONALE AND TECHNIQUES FOR ENTERAL NUTRITION

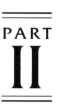

PART II

A Successful Technique for Providing Enteral Nutrition

CHAPTER 6

Bradley C. Borlase, M.D., M.S.,
Stacey J. Bell, M.S., R.D.,
R. Armour Forse, M.D., Ph.D.,
and George L. Blackburn, M.D., Ph.D.

INTRODUCTION

Nutritional support is an important adjunctive treatment for the hospitalized patient. Malnutrition is associated with an increase in complications, length of stay, and cost (1). It is unfortunate that the majority of malnutrition today is either not identified or ignored, even though it occurs in 25–50% of hospitalized patients (2,3). A recent study has shown that recognition and treatment of malnutrition will reduce length of stay by 25%, which may have been attributed to the use of a specific enteral product (4). However, other data indicate that such reductions may result simply from early recognition and treatment of the malnutrition (5).

Current nutritional therapies for malnutrition include specialized nutrition support as total parenteral nutrition (TPN) and as enteral nutrition (EN) by tube. While TPN remains an important therapeutic option, the American Society for Parenteral and Enteral Nutrition recommends that "if the gut works, use it" (6). Indeed, EN has not been isolated to use only for patients not in the intensive care unit (ICU) alone, but has been shown to be efficacious in critically ill patients as well (7,8). It is clear that the most expensive EN formula still costs less than TPN in the vast majority of patients (i.e., non-ICU) (9). The concept of using EN in conjunction with TPN as "metabolic support" rather than solely as nutritional support has recently become popular.

Metabolic support involves the provision of calories for the preservation of structures and function rather than the restoration of lean body mass and fat stores (11). Enteral diets used to provide metabolic support therefore typically tend to have a low calorie to nitrogen ratio (<100). Combined feeding provides additional benefits as well (12). Enteral feeding may favorably influence both immunologic and metabolic problems due to injury, surgery, or disease by down-regulating responses to inflammatory challenges (13).

This chapter summarizes the technique used at the New England Deaconess Hospital (Boston, MA) by the Enteral Nutrition Service (ENS). The hospital maintains both a Nutrition Support Service (NSS), which is consulted for TPN as well as tube feeding, and an Enteral Nutrition Service, which is consulted strictly for enterally fed patients (14). The primary advantages of the ENS methods include ease of application, high tolerance rates, low diarrhea rates, general applicability to both critically ill and non-critical patients, and cost effectiveness. This is not to imply that there is no role for TPN. Instead, TPN and EN complement each other and the future of specialized nutrition support is to match these two complementary modes of feeding.

PATIENT SELECTION CRITERIA

There are only four major contraindications to enteral nutrition: bowel obstruction, shock, >90% small bowel resection, and mesenteric ischemia (6). Patients admitted with bowel obstruction are at high risk for malnutrition and should receive TPN until surgery, at which time a feeding catheter may be placed. Combined nutritional support can be administered postoperatively although patients should be stabilized; they should be normotensive without pressor support before beginning enteral nutrition.

Patients with minimal or no small bowel (<10%) should not be considered for enteral feeding. However, it is imperative to document the length of small bowel, since many patients with so-called "short bowel" are incorrectly assigned to receive nothing by mouth (NPO). Bowel function may eventually adapt to intestinal feedings for full nutritional support.

Physicians should be aware of a subset of patients with profound vascular disease who may not tolerate enteral feedings except slowly over an extended period. Total parenteral nutrition or combined feeding with low volumes of enteral feedings (e.g., 10 ml/hr) may be administered for this rare subset of patients. Over 2–3 weeks, the enteral feeding is slowly advanced and TPN weaned. This allows the bowel to adapt to enteral support.

WHEN TO START EN

Enteral nutrition may be initiated at any time during hospitalization if no contraindications exist. It should preferably be started as soon as possible following admission or surgery. In postoperative patients, we begin tube feeding within 12 hr after surgery, usually in the recovery room. This enhances reservation of gastrointestinal tract mucos, thus improving tolerance and decreasing diarrhea (15).

FORMULA SELECTION

Although myriad enteral formulas exist, they can be classified in two general varieties: monomeric (elemental) and polymeric (16). Elemental diets contain predigested macronutrients, while polymeric diets have nutrients in an intact state. Both contain all known essential micronutrients in 1,000–2,500 ml. Jones et al. have shown no significant differences in tolerance and/or diarrhea rates between these two types of enteral diets in randomized, prospective trials (17). However, the patients they studied had no gastrointestinal impairment, were nonstressed, and had serum albumin concentrations of 3.6 g/dl. Moreover, serum albumin levels are of no importance in tolerance or the decision to use enteral diets (18,19), despite a theoretical advantage of elemental diets in patients with profoundly low serum albumin levels (<2.5) (20); our experience and that of others (21) does not corroborate this advantage.

We are currently prospectively randomizing patients to receive elemental or polymeric diets, irrespective of severity of illness or albumin level. There does not appear to be a significant difference in tolerance, but the results are pending. Therefore, we would recommend starting patients on a polymeric diet. However, patients who are fed intragastrically and have a high severity of illness should receive low-fat (<10 g/L) elemental diets because of the problems associated with the aspiration of fat.

FEEDING TUBE SELECTION

Many types of feeding catheters are also available, ranging from needle catheter jejunostomies, pediatric feeding tubes (e.g., #5 Fr), or large-bore (>#12 Fr) gastrostomies (e.g., Foley). The needle catheter jejunostomy has been shown to be highly successful in young trauma patients and patients with cancer who have a low severity of illness (15). We have found that these tubes have a high failure rate (dislodgement, clogging) in geriatric and/or chronically ill patients who may require prolonged feeding, particularly after a period of acute ICU illness.

We do not routinely use the stomach as a feeding conduit due to emptying problems secondary to severity of illness and comorbid disease (e.g., diabetes). The acute-phase response associated with many infectious states appears to be mediated by interleukin-1. When recombinant interleukin-1 was administered to rats fed a liquid diet, delayed gastric emptying occurred (22). Nasoduodenal and nasojejunal feeding tubes offer an advantage over nasogastric feeding, but there are problems with sinus infection and patient discomfort and/or dislodgement. Gastroduodenal and gastrojejunal feeding tubes are an improvement, in that they eliminate nasal intubation, but they are still associated with pyloric erosions and retrograde progression of the tube tip, causing infusion of formula into the stomach or upper levels of the duodenum and thus stimulating the pancreas.

Our experience with enteral feeding has led us to use primarily a jejunal feeding catheter except in cases of profound immunosuppression (e.g., liver transplantation, acquired immunodeficiency syndrome, inflammatory bowel). In these cases, a nasojejunal tube may be substituted. This technique enables the patient to receive a full complement of calories and protein quickly, starting immediately, and achieving goal rates by day 4 with minimal gastric emptying problems or stimulation of the duodenal–pancreatic axis.

To utilize the jejunal feeding tube indefinitely as a conduit for nutrition and medications, we currently use a biliary T-tube modified as Mangot's early common duct tube placed 18–24 inches from the ligament of Treitz via purse-string sutures. This is described in detil in Chapter 11. This creates direct access to the small bowel, eliminating the Weitzel technique. If this tube becomes unusable due to dislodgement, clogging, leakage), a new catheter may thus be placed at the bedside. In addition, this technique has the lowest complication rate, particularly when used in the critically ill geriatric patient (19,23).

STRENGTH OF FORMULA AND RATE OF INFUSION

The vast majority of patients may be started on full-strength formulas at infusion rates of 10 ml/hr as soon as possible after surgery or admission. Advancement should be 10 ml/hr every 12–24 hr until all nutrient requirements are met. Most patients fed with total EN receive 50–60 ml/hr (18), and all patients except those with >30% body burns or significant head trauma are maintained on 25–30 kCal/kg and 1.5g/protein/kg (24). Therefore, patients started on postpyloric EN (best results with jejunal feeding) should reach their full nutritional requirements with

4–5 days, eliminating the need for central access except to manage fluid, acid–base, and electrolyte balance.

ADVANCEMENT FROM ACUTE TO CHRONIC CARE

Patients successfully tolerating full EN may be quickly advanced (usually 5–7 days) to night-cycled feedings, allowing patients freedom of movement during waking hours. Complete nutritional requirements are given over a 12-hr period, which requires doubling the hourly rate of delivery of the formula. With the use of cycled feedings, patients may be discharged from the hospital earlier, since attainment of oral nutritional goals is no longer mandatory for discharge. This is especially true among elderly patients, who often require a prolonged convalescent period to regain adequate oral intake. Usually after 60–90 days at home or in a rehabilitation facility, the older patient is able to maintain an adequate oral intake, and the feeding tube may be removed. The enterocutaneous fistula closes quickly, usually in 3–5 days.

REFERENCES

1. Smith P, Smith A, Toan B: Nutritional Care Arts, Private Pay Days. Chicago: Nutrition Care Management Institute, 1989.
2. Bistrian BR, Blackburn GL, Vitale J, Cochran D, Naylor J: Prevalence of malnutrition in general medical patients. JAMA 235:1557–1560, 1976.
3. Bistrian BR, Blackburn GL, Hallowell E, Heddle R: Protein status of general surgical patients. JAMA 230:858–860, 1974.
4. Daly JW, Lieberman M, Goldfine J, Shoni J, Weintraub N, Rosato EF, Lavin P: Enteral nutrition with supplemental arginine, RNA, and omega-3 fatty acids; a prospective clinical trial. JPEN 15:19S, 1991.
5. Seltzer MH, Slocum BA, Cataldi-Betcher EL, Fileti C, Gerson N: Instant nutritional assessment: absolute weight loss and surgical mortality. JPEN 6:218–221, 1982.
6. ASPEN Board of Directors: Guidelines for the use of enteral nutrition in the adult patient. JPEN 11:435–439, 1987.
7. Kelly TWJ, Patrick MR, Hillman KM. Study of diarrhea in critically ill patients. Crit Care Med 11:7–9, 1983.
8. Pesola GE, Hogg JE, Yonnios, T, McConnell RE, Carlon GC. Isotonic nasogastric tube feedings: do they cause diarrhea? Crit Care Med 17:1151–1155, 1989.
9 Szeluga DJ, Stuart RK, Brookmeyer R, Utermohlen V, Santos GW: Nutrition support of bone marrow transplant recipients: a prospective, randomized clinical trial comparing total parenteral nutrition to an enteral feeding program. Cancer Res 47:3309–3316, 1987.

10. Bower RH, Talamini MA, Sax HC, Hamilton F, Fisher JE. Postoperative enteral vs. parenteral nutrition. Arch Surg 121:1040–1045, 1986.
11. Cerra FB: Hypermetabolic organ failure, and metabolic support. Surgery 101:1–14, 1987.
12. Borlase BC, Babineau TJ, Forse RA, Bell SJ, Blackburn GL: Enteral nutritional support, in Rippe JM, Irwin RS, Alpert JS, Dalen JE, Fink M (eds) Intensive Care Medicine, pp. 1669–1691, 1991.
13. Lowry SF: The route of feeding influences injury responses. J Trauma 30:S10–S15, 1990.
14. Borlase B, Bell SJ, Swails W, Bistrain BR, Dascoulias K, Forse RA, et al: Rationale and efficacy of an enteral service. Presented at the ASPEN Clinical Congress, San Francisco, CA, January 29, 1990; abstract 26.
15. Jones TN, Moore FA, Moore EE, McCroskey BL: Gastrointestinal symptoms attributed to jejunostomy feeding after major abdominal trauma—a critical analysis. Crit Care Med 17:1146–1150, 1989.
16. Bell SJ, Pasulka PS, Blackburn GL: Enteral formulas, in Skipper A (ed) Dietitian's Handbook of Enteral and Parenteral Nutrition. Rockville, MD: ASPEN Publishers, 1989, pp. 279–292.
17. Jones BJM, Lees R, Andrews J, Frost P, Silk DBA: Comparison of an elemental and polymeric enteral diets in patients with normal gastrointestinal function. Gut 24:78–84, 1983.
18. Patterson ML, Dominguez JM, Lyman B, Cuddy PG, Pemberton LB: Enteral feeding in the hypoalbuminemic patient. JPEN 14:362–365, 1990.
19. Borlase BC, Bell SJ, Lewis EJ, Swails W, Bistrian BR, Forse RA, et al: Tolerance to enteral tube feeding diets in hypoalbuminemic critically ill, geriatric patients: a prospective randomized trial. Surg Obstet Gynecol 174:181–188, 1992.
20. Brinson RR, Kolts BE. Hypoalbuminemia as an indicator of diarrhea incidence in critically ill patients. Crit Care Med 15:506–509, 1987.
21. Gottschlich MM, Warden GD, Michel M, Haven P, Kopcha R, Jenkins M, et al. Diarrhea in tube-fed burn patients: incidence, etiology, nutritional impact, and prevention. JPEN 12:338–345, 1988.
22. Nompleggi D, Teo TC, Blackburn GL, Bistrian BR: Human recombinant interleukin-1 decreases gastric emptying in the rat. Gastroenterology 94:A326, 1988.
23. Khoury T, Borlase BC, Forse RA, Bell SJ, Blackburn GL, Bistrian BR: Associated complications using a feeding jejunostromy in hospitalized patients. In preparation, 1991.
24. Shanbhogue LKR, Chwals WJ, Weintraub M, Blackburn GL, Bistrian BR: Parenteral nutrition in the surgical patient. Br J Surg 74:172–180, 1987.

Development of an Enteral Nutrition Support Service

CHAPTER 7

Stacey J. Bell, M.S., R.D.,
Bradley C. Borlase, M.D., M.S.,
Wendy Swails, R.D., CNSD,
Kathy Dascoulias, D.T.R.,
and R. Armour Forse, M.D., Ph.D.

BACKGROUND

During the early 1970s, two classic reports identified the prevalence of malnutrition among medical and surgical patients in an urban, teaching hospital (1,2). Medical patients had at least a 44% incidence of malnutrition according to a variety of standard assessment parameters, including anthropometric measurements, serum albumin concentrations, and hematocirt (1). Half of the surgical patients surveyed were malnourished as demonstrated by similar measures (2).

At about the same time, Dudrick and colleagues (3) perfected the technique of feeding via the superior vena cava, known today as total parenteral nutrition (TPN). This method allowed for provision of hypertonic dextrose, protein, fats, and all known essential micronutrients. This represented the first instance in which clinicians could use a dependable means to aliment critically ill patients by vein. Of course, as with any treatment, risks were involved, predominantly those problems associated with line insertion (e.g., pneumothorax), thrombosis, line sepsis, and metabolic complications associated with the feeding itself (e.g., hyperglycemia).

Given the prevalence of the malnourishment and the discovery of a reliable means for correcting the problem, the use of TPN rapidly became the most common form of nutritional support. However, it also became apparent that there was more to TPN than line insertion and solution delivery. Numerous problems arose that required correction by a multidisciplinary array of staff members. Nurses specially trained in the insertion and maintenance of intravenous (i.v.) lines were required to monitor catheter care. Highly skilled dietitians were required to assess patients' nutritional status and needs, first to determine who should receive TPN and subsequently to calculate nutrient needs. Specialized pharmacists were needed to produce the formulas and advise physicians as to which drugs could be mixed in the TPN formulas. This need for diverse skills led to the creation of a formal team approach to caring for patients receiving TPN.

Many authors (4–7) have identified that patients managed by such a team approach have had fewer complications. Reports of fewer catheter-related complication (4–6), more frequent performance of nutritional assessments (4), and better compliance with prescribed nutritional goals (4) have been made for team-managed patients. As a result, nutrition support teams sprang up through the country; in 1983 there were estimated to be 521 teams nationwide (7).

During the late 1980s and into the early 1990s, intense interest grew in enteral nutrition support. Although clearly a more physiological means of alimenting the patient, enteral support is also less costly (8). Some investigators have theorized that immune function is improved through stimulation of gut hormones (9). Moreover, gut integrity is preserved by enteral feeding, suggesting that a healthy gut would be impermeable to indigenous gut flora, and endotoxemia thus prevented (10). New enteral food components have recently become available that may even strengthen the gastrointestinal mucosa (glutamine) (11) or stimulate the immune system (arginine, fish oil, and RNA nucleotides), leading to fewer postoperative complications and shorted stay (12). Many of these new food components are unavailable parenterally.

WHY THE ENS WAS FORMED

Despite the remarkable technical achievements in TPN, relatively few advances have been made in enteral nutrition, making it a less dependable means of alimentation, particularly in the intensive care unit (ICU). Recently, however, we (13) described a successful technique to feed critically ill patients in the ICU: feed postpylorically, beyond the ligament of Trietz; begin administration of the formula early, within 24 hr postoperatively or soon after admission for medical patients; infuse formula slowly, beginning at 10 ml/hr at full strength, and increase daily by 10 ml/hr; and select a low-fat, elemental formula until goal rate is achieved and then switch to a polymeric formula. These methods were validated in a randomized, prospective trial in which we enterally alimented critically ill patients with mean serum albumin concentrations of 2.3 g/dl (14). Both elemental diets used in the trial were successfully administered and tolerated, which sparked increased interest by the surgical house staff in providing enteral nutrition.

Yet with the increased use of enteral feeding, new complications not seen before developed. These may have been due to the inexperience of residents and house staff in using enteral nutrition, to the increased severity of illness of the patients receiving enteral nutrition, or to a combination of both. Also, there are new specialized formulas with unique uses and a multitude of additives, especially for the critically ill patient. For example, given the complexity of care rendered to these patients, we found that physicians were ordering numerous medications via the feeding tube since many patients no longer needed intravenous access: this sequence of events resulted in more frequently clogged feeding tubes. The Enteral Nutrition Service (ENS), still in an early stage of development, worked with surgeons who gradually began to place larger tubes at the time of surgery if they placed them at all. Indeed, the ENS remained frustrated knowing that enteral feeding could be successfully used in these patients, of whom many were supported totally intravenously during their critical phase of illness.

Other complications arose because metabolic management of these patients was more difficult and often beyond the scope of practice of dietitians, who were responsible for nutritional care. Organizers of the ENS began to be queried by the dietitians regarding means of care. In addition, amid the conduct of several clinical enteral protocols, no system existed for accruing patients in an efficient manner.

At this point, the ENS formally split off from the 18-year-old Nutrition Support Team, representing perhaps the first dedicated ENS in the country. Others (15) have identified that a traditional nutritional support service managed both enteral and TPN patients.

Using experience gained during the creation of the TPN-oriented nutrition support team, the ENS was designed to be multidisciplinary. The team was codirected by two staff surgeons (BCB and RAF) who have research and clinical interest in enteral feeding; an "on-call" schedule was devised for monthly coverage between the two. The ENS employs a dietitian as the administrator (SJB), and the inpatient clinical staff of dietitians (n = 5) actively participate as does one clinical dietetic technician. Team rounds are held daily (except Tuesday).

DAILY ACTIVITIES

The ENS is presently available to assist with any surgical patient who is receiving a tube feeding diet and who does not receive TPN. The ENS is consulted in the usual fashion, through the physician's order sheet (Figure 7-1). Eligible patients may also be referred through the Nutrition Support Team, which turns over stable patients who are to be tube fed after the use of TPN is completed.

After a consultation is received, the on-call ENS surgeon responds in the Consult Section of the medical record. These consults are currently billed under the CPT code of Extended Level of Service (90610). Each consultation is accompanied by a formal nutritional assessment, which is performed by the dietetic technician (Figure 7-2). Classification of the degree and type of malnutrition is required for billing purposes.

Each staff dietitian is responsible for the daily care of ENS patients on floors normally covered and reports at rounds on compliance and tolerance to the tube feeding regimen and on new developments. The team reviews the current information and makes suggestions to assist the dietitian, with notes in the progress section of medical records. All notes are cowritten with the on-call ENS surgeon. Before the ENS was formed, the staff dietitians expressed frustration that the notes were not being implemented. Since the jointly written notes have begun, this problem has been greatly reduced, although one of the ENS physicians must sometimes still contact the patient's physician in person. Depending on the patient's degree of clinical stability, notes are written on 2–3 days per week, with more stable patients having joint notes twice a week (Figure 7-1). Only notes that are jointly written may be billed. However, given that the system based on diagnosis-related groups (DRGs) is in place in Massachusetts, the ENS is likely only to receive money from patients who have private insurance. The ENS is now evaluating 8 patients and receives 0.85 new consults daily.

JUSTIFICATION

Since its inception, the ENS has improved the quality of care while reducing hospital costs. Patient care was improved by the ENS primarily through careful metabolic management and efficient discharge planning. Moreover, the surgeons run the rounds as a teaching mileu for dietitians. During rounds, the patients' clinical status are thoroughly reviewed and, given the high severity of illness, many metabolic abnormalities can be discussed. The ENS notes describe appropriate choices for therapy and the correct administration route. For example, the ENS has shown that medications and electrolytes are put in the tube feeding when they should have been administered intravenously. If the patient has no venous access, the ENS instructs the physician and nurse on how to avoid iatrogenic side effects; the ENS may recommend that a patient who requires 60 mEq sodium chloride daily receive it as a split dose of 20 mEq three times daily.

Another aspect of improved quality of patient care includes tolerance to feeding regimen. Diarrhea has been reported to be the most frequent complication of

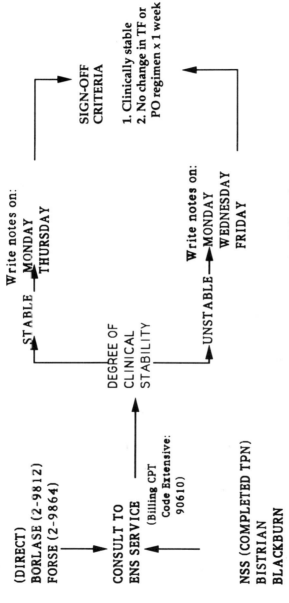

Figure 7-1. Decision tree of how the enteral nutrition support service (ENS) works.

ASSESSMENT OF NUTRITIONAL STATUS FOR PATIENTS RECEIVING ENTERAL TUBE FEEDING DIETS

NUTRITION SUPPORT SERVICE
NEW ENGLAND DEACONESS HOSPITAL

ANTHROPOMETRIC MEASUREMENTS

Height _____ cm _____ inches

Present weight _____ kg _____ pounds _____ % ideal weight _____ % weight loss in last 3 months _____

Usual weight _____ kg _____ pounds _____ % ideal weight _____ date

Ideal weight _____ kg _____ pounds

BMI _____ $\dfrac{\text{Weight (kg)}}{\text{Height}^2 \text{ (m)}}$

BIOCHEMICAL INDICES

<u>Urine</u>

Ideal Creatinine _____ (mg) (Ideal Males = 23 mg xIBW)
(Females = 18 mg x IBW)

Date: ___/___/___ Actual Creatinine _____ (mg)

		Severe	Moderate	Mild
Creatinine Height Index	_____ %	<60%	60-80%	-
Urinary Urea Nitrogen	_____ gm	-	-	-
Nitrogen Balance	_____ gm	-	-	-
Catabolic Index	_____ gm	>5 gm	0-5 gm	<0 g
Total dietary nitrogen	_____ gm	-	-	-

<u>Serum</u>

Date: ___/___/___

Albumin	_____ gm/dl	< 2.5	2.5-3.0	3.0-3.5
Total lymphocyte count	_____ cell/mm³	<800	800-1200	-

<u>Summary</u> (check one box)

Other Protein-Calorie Malnutrition (Not depleted but stressed or septic) ICD-9 Code 263.8 weight loss < 5% albumin > 3.2 g/dL anticipate prolonged LOS	Nutritional Marasmus ICD-9 Code 261 weight loss ≥ 10% albumin > 3.2 g/dL	Kwashiorkor (Hypoalbuminemia) ICD-9 Code 260 weight loss ≤ 10% albumin ≤ 3.2 g/dL
Mixed Marasmus-Hypoalbuminemia Malnutrition of mild degree ICD-9 Code 263.1 25% ≤ weight loss > 10% albumin ≤ 3.2 g/dL	Mixed Marasmus Hypoalbuminemia Malnutrition of Moderate Degree ICD-9 Code 263.0 40% ≤ weight loss > 25% albumin ≤ 3.2 g/dL	Obesity ICD-9 Code 278.0 BMI > 30

Figure 7-2. Assessment of nutritional status for patients receiving enteral tube feeding diets.

tube feeding, with rates as high as 40–60% (16). However, in a recent study conducted in critically ill patients receiving enteral diets, we found no diarrhea (14). The ENS addresses diarrhea and signs of all intolerance to tube feeding at the onset of symptoms, thus avoiding complications that could lead to cessation of the enteral diet.

DIAGNOSIS:

ENERGY AND PROTEIN REQUIREMENTS

BASAL ENERGY EXPENDITURE (BEE) by Harris-Benedict Equation

Males: $66 + (13.8 \times W) + (5 \times H) - (6.8 \times A)$ W = actual wt. in kg
                                                                                            H = height in cm
Females: $665 + (9.6 \times W) + (1.8 \times H) - (4.7 \times A)$ A = age in years

     BEE = _____ Actual Weight (____ kg)
     BEE = _____ Ideal Weight (____ kg)

ENERGY REQUIREMENTS

Anabolic requirements:

BEE x 1.2 - 1.3 = _____

BEE x 1.3 - 1.4 = _____

Maintenance Requirements
BEE x 1.2 = _____

ICU Ventilator Dependent Patient
    a. Empiric Formula =
       REE = 22 x W
    b. Multiple Linear Regression =
REE = $613 + (19.7 \times W) - (525.6 \times Sex) + (28.7 \times WBC)$

Where: W = actual wt. in kg
              WBC = White cell count in 1000 cells/mm^3
              Male = 1
              Female = 2

Measured Resting Energy Expenditure =

     Kcal/24 hours = _____

Estimated Energy Expenditure (EEE) =
(Based on 24 Hour Urinary Creatinine Level)
EEE = $964 + (0.488 \times mg$ Urinary Creatinine)
    EEE = _____

Hernandez Formula*
Kcal goal = 1.04 BEE - 68 kcal
    Kcal goal = _____
* based on 28 patients; mean age was 69±8 yrs
(using lowest weight, admission or actual)
In preparation, 1992.

CARBOHYDRATE REQUIREMENTS

2.5 - 4 mg/kg/min = _____ g

PROTEIN REQUIREMENTS

Anabolic (1.5 g/kg Ideal wt.) = _____

Maintenance (1.2 g/kg Ideal wt.) = _____

Discharge from NSS (date and reason) - specify present diet order.

Figure 7-2. (Continued).

The ENS recommendations have also resulted in financial savings. Frequently, the ENS recommends change from a more costly formula to a less costly one that is nutritionally equivalent. In addition, some patients are overfed, and a reduction in total volume is advised. Polypharmacy frequently plagues tube-fed patients. We frequently question the need for drug, electrolyte, and vitamin additives that are no longer required but have not been removed from medication orders. The ENS has encountered patients receiving multiple doses of antidiarrheals when one would suffice, and inexpensive oral electrolytes are recommended to replace the more expensive parenteral form.

Patients who received jejunostomy feeding tubes can be discharged sooner because they do not need to be able to consume all their nutrients orally. Patients are discharged on night-cycle tube feedings, which ENS recommends early in the course of care. Thus, calorie counts for the oral diet can be obtained at home and be reviewed by the dietitian when the patient has an appointment with his or her surgeon.

SUMMARY

Just as nutrition support teams resulted from intense interest in TPN, enteral nutrition services are likely to follow suit. Enteral feeding is a cost-effective means of alimentation and can be successfully administered to the most critically ill patient. Its use will undoubtedly reduce medical costs while enhancing patient care.

REFERENCES

1. Bistrian BR, Blackburn GL, Vitale J, Cochhran D, Naylor J: Prevalence of malnutrition in general medical patients. JAMA 235:1557–1560, 1976.
2. Bistrian BR, Blackburn GL, Hallowell E, Heddle R: Protein status of general surgical patients. JAMA 230:858–860, 1974.
3. Dudrick SJ, Wilmore DW, Vars HM, Rhoads JR: Long-term total parenteral nutrition with growth, development and positive nitrogen balance. Surgery 64:134–142, 1968.
4. Traeger SM, Williams GB, Milliren G, Young DS, Fisher M, Haug MT: Total parenteral nutrition by a nutrition support team: improved quality of care. JPEN 10:408–412, 1986.
5. Nehme AE: Nutrition support of the hospitalized patient. JAMA 243:1906–1908, 1980.
6. Faubion WC, Wesley J, Khalidi N, Silva J: Total parenteral nutrition catheter sepsis: impact of the team approach. JPEN 10:642–645, 1986.
7. McShane CM, Fox HM: Nutrition support teams—a 1983 survey. JPEN 9:263–268, 1985.
8. Bower RH, Talamini MA, Sax HC, Hamilton F, Fischer JE: Postoperative enteral versus parenteral nutrition. Arch Surg 121:1040–1045, 1986.
9. Lowry SF: The route of feeding influences injury responses. J Trauma 30:S10–S15, 1990.
10. Deitch EA: Bacterial translocation of the gut flora. J. Trauma 30:S184–S188, 1990.

11. Souba WW, Smith RJ, Wilmore DW: Glutamine metabolism by the intestinal tract. JPEN 9:608–617, 1985.
12. Daly JM, Lieberman M, Goldfine J, Shou J, Weintraub FN, Rosato EF, Lavin P: Enteral nutrition with supplemental arginine, RNA, and omega-3 fatty acids: a prospective clinical trial. JPEN 15:19S (abst 17), 1991.
13. Borlase BC, Babineau TJ, Forse RA, Bell SJ, Blackburn GL: Enteral nutrition support, in Rippe JM, Irwin RS, Alpert JS, Dalen JE, Fink M (eds) Intensive Care Medicine, 1991. 2nd ed Little Brown & Co., Boston 1991.
14. Borlase BC, Bell SJ, Lewis EJ, Swails W, Bistrian BR, Forse RA, Blackburn GL: Tolerance to enteral tube feeding diets in hypoalbuminemic critically ill, geriatric patients: a prospective randomized trial. Surg Gynecol Obstet., 1991. SGO 1992; 174:181–188.
15. Powers DA, Brown RO, Cowan GS, Luther RW, Sutherland DA, Drexler PG: Nutritional support team versus non-team management of enteral nutritional support in a Veteran's Administration Medical Center Teaching Hospital. JPEN 10:635–638, 1986.
16. Pesola GE, Hogg JE, Yonnios T, McConnell RE, Carlon GC: Isotonic nasogastric tube feedings: do they cause diarrhea? Crit Care Med 17:1151–1155, 1989.

CHAPTER 8

Early Postoperative Feeding

Todd N. Jones, M.S., R.N., CNSN,
Ernest E. Moore, M.D.,
and Frederick A. Moore, M.D.

INTRODUCTION

Nutritional support of the acutely stressed patient has long been recognized as a major component of surgical care. Severe trauma, burns, and sepsis are characterized by a hypermetabolic, hypercatabolic response that rapidly depletes vital nutrient reserves. The extraordinary demand for energy erodes lean body mass, depletes visceral protein stores, and compromises immune function, setting the stage for postoperative complications, multiple organ failure, and death. This chapter focuses on the pathophysiology of stress-related malnutrition, employing the multisystem-injured patient as a clinical example for aggressive nutritional support.

HISTORICAL PERSPECTIVE

Despite many important advances in the early 20th century, only in the past 30 years has nutritional support been technically feasible and clinically available for improving patient care. Enteral nutrition employing intubation of various portions of the gastrointestinal (GI) tract has a long, but sporadic history dating to the ancient Egyptians (1). Nutrient enemas were used before the birth of Christ and were commonplace in the 1890s until Edsal and Miller (2) demonstrated that rectally administered protein was eliminated essentially unabsorbed. In fact, President Garfield was treated with rectal instillation of whiskey and beef protein in an attempt to provide nourishment while he was unsuccessfully treated for an abdominal gunshot wound (1). Various techniques for surgical access of the upper GI tract for nutritional supplementation were introduced in the late 1800s. Surmay, in 1878, performed the first surgical jejunostomy (3). In 1892, Maydl (4) devised the first continent jejunostomy based on a Roux-en-Y jejunal loop. Different techniques of gastrostomy tube placement for the administration of nutrition were exemplified by Witzel in 1891, Stamm in 1894, and Janeway in 1913 (5). Problems with leakage and obstruction, however, prevented these techniques from gaining wide acceptance. Transnasal intubation for feeding was popularized in the early part of this century because of the significant morbidity associated with the surgically placed tubes. Andressen (6), in 1918, is credited with one of the earliest attempts at nasojejunal feeding in patients undergoing gastrointestinal operations. Abbott and Rawsen (7), in the late 1930s advanced the concept of using a double-lumen tube, providing both gastric decompression and access for jejunal feeding. Moss et al. (8), pursuing this concept, added a third lumen to vent esophageal air in an effort to ameliorate postoperative ileus. Although transnasal tubes eliminated intraperitoneal complications, the earlier large tubes were associated with rhinitis, pharyngitis, and otitis, as well as gastroesophageal sphincter incompetence leading to reflux and aspiration. The modern era of enteral feeding began in the 1950s with the development of small-bore polyethylene catheters for nasoenteric as well as direct transjejunal feeding. MacDonald (9) was the early pioneer in the 1950s, while Delany et al. (10) devised the currently used jejunal feeding catheter about a decade ago. The safety of this advanced technique has been corroborated by the subsequent extensive clinical work of Page et al. (11).

The first attempts at parenteral infusion of nutrients followed shortly after the discovery of circulation in 1616 by William Harvey (12). Franaseo Felli and Christopher Wren demonstrated a successful intravenous infusion of ale, wine, and opium in dogs in the mid–1650s (13). Shortly thereafter, Richard Lowen and Sir Edward King recorded the first transfusion in humans using sheep's blood (14). In the 1870s the six major dietary components (water, salt, vitamins, carbohydrates, fat, and protein) were recognized. Sterility became recognized as essential for intravenous infusion in the 1890s and saline, as well as sugar, solutions were used to treat shock. Roswell Park (15), in 1907, described a technique of intravenous administration of fluid using a funnel, rubber tubing, and venous cutdown for vascular access.

Alimentation by the parenteral route began to be developed in the early 1900s. In 1913, Henrique (16) infused a protein hydrosylate of goat muscle into dogs and claimed to produced nitrogen balance. Cuthbertson's description of the hypermetabolic response to injury was made in 1930, documenting obligatory muscle wasting and increased oxygen consumption as characteristic of the stress response. He demonstrated that feeding an injured patient with high-quality protein and adequate calories tended to minimize weight loss but did not reduce the elevated urinary nitrogen excretion associated with major injury (17). Elman (18), in the late 1930s, demonstrated the first successful delivery of intravenous (IV) protein in humans. He infused an enzymatic hydrolysate of casein and pancreas (Amigen). W.C. Rose (19), in 1937, is credited with isolating the eight essential amino acids in humans. Rose and his co-workers determined the minimal daily requirement of each essential amino acid to maintain nitrogen equilibrium. This research paved the way for the introduction of FreAmine, the first crystalline amino acid solution, in 1971. Fat emulsions were developed in the 1930s but were considered unstable. In 1951, commercially prepared fat emulsions produced positive nitrogen balance but were associated with a high incidence of complications including anemia, bleeding, and fat embolism. Not until 1975 did a safe and effective IV lipid solution (Intralipid) become available in the United States.

The modern era of total parenteral nutrition (TPN) by central vein began with the classic work of Rhode et al. (20), who were able to maintain adult dogs exclusively on venous nutrition for 141 days. This continuous central venous infusion was first used in patients in 1961, but the massive volumes necessary to deliver adequate nutrition required liberal use of diuretics. In 1968, Dudrick and colleagues (21) demonstrated normal growth and development in beagle puppies fed exclusively by the intravenous route, which led to human trials in which the efficacy of TPN was demonstrated.

The past 20 years has seen a plethora of research in nutritional support practice. There has been considerable changes in recommended doses of calories, protein, and other nutrients. The development of disease-specific formulations, nutrient modulators, and growth factors has set the stage for continued investigation of nutritional management, especially in the critically ill patient.

INJURY STRESS RESPONSE

The metabolic response to injury teleologically optimizes the internal environment for survival as well as wound repair. This complex but coordinated reaction maximizes oxygen delivery to vital organs while it mobilizes substrate from dispensable supportive tissue. The injury stress response (hypermetabolism/hypercatabolism) has been well characterized physiologically, but the intricate driving mechanism is being redefined continuously. The neuroendocrine component has been recognized for decades; the activated hypothalmic–pituitary–adrenal axis produces elevated plasma levels of catecholamines, glucocorticoids, and glucagon. Wilmore et al. (22), infusing various combinations of these counterregulatory hormones into healthy volunteers, have documented a synergistic interaction reproducing the hypermetabolism observed following major trauma. However, the same triple-hormone infusion does not provoke the hypercatabolism observed clinically, implicating other factors as responsible for the obligatory proteolysis of critical illness (23). Indeed, metabolic research over the past decade has concentrated on the cell-to-cell interaction, yielding a multitude of inflammatory mediators: activated complement, cyclo-oxygenase products, lipoxygenase products, toxic oxygen metabolites, neutrophil proteases, platelet-activating factor, and various cytokines. Although interleukin-1 (IL-1) and tumor necrosis factor (TNF) are presently considered the primary signals of protein breakdown (24,25), there appear to be other critical elements (26). Thus, the postinjury stress response is the net result of a complex interdependent cascade consisting of cell-generated inflammatory mediators as well as neuromediated counterregulatory hormones.

SUBSTRATE DEMANDS

The effects of the activated macro- and microendocrine systems are additive, and the corresponding rise in energy expenditure relates to the magnitude as well as injury mechanism. Energy expenditure typically increases 80–100% following major burns, 40–50% following closed head injury, and 30–40% following multisystem trauma. Net somatic muscle proteolysis occurs as protein catabolism exceeds synthesis (27). Carcass protein stores are mobilized to support the more critical visceral organs. The branched-chain amino acids (leucine, isoleucine, and valine) become important oxidative fuels for skeletal muscle, heart, and brain (28,29). The glucogenic amino acids, principally alanine, are taken up by the liver to produce greater quantities of glucose while glutamine becomes the preferred oxidative fuel for the gastrointestinal tract as well as the immune system (30). Circulating amino acids also provide critical substrate for hepatic acute phase protein synthesis, wound healing, and maintenance of other vital organ function (31,32). Carbohydrate metabolism is characterized by a persistent, hepatic gluconeogenesis that is not suppressed by exogenous administration of glucose or insulin (33). Abnormal glucose tolerance exists, evidenced by high serum glucose concentrations, but insulin levels are normal or even elevated. Overall glucose utilization is elevated due to increased demands by the central nervous and hematopoietic systems as well as injured tissue, while clearance by skeletal muscle and adipose tissue is blunted. The kinetics of fat metabolism following injury are less well defined. Lipolysis is enhanced, free fatty acid oxidation is accelerated, and ketosis suppressed (34,35). The typical postinjury decline in respiratory quotient (RQ) corroborates that fat is a major source of energy during this stress period (36), but controversy remains as to the "preferred oxidative fuel."

Hypercatabolism is a prominent feature of the early postinjury stress response. The obligatory rate of protein turnover generally parallels the rise in metabolic rate following trauma, with the notable exception of high spinal cord injury (37). The ultimate fate of catabolized amino acid carbon skeletons is energy production via the Krebs cycle, while ammonia is detoxified as reflected in the urinary excretion of urea nitrogen. Patients sustaining multisystem trauma generally lose 13–18 g nitrogen per day and, if compounded by closed head injury with increased intracranial pressure or major long bone and pelvic fractures, nitrogen excretion frequently exceeds 25 g daily.

METABOLIC ASSESSMENT AND RISK STRATIFICATION

Nutritional assessment of the acutely injured patient is essential, both to identify the need for aggressive nutritional support and to ascertain its efficacy. The recognition of malnutrition as a common problem in hospitalized patients has stimulated the development of nutritional assessment profiles. These profiles, designed primarily for patients with chronic malnourished states, can be useful in the acutely injured patient both to determine baseline status and monitor continuing nutritional requirements. Metabolic assessment of the injured patients is outlined in Table 8-1. Our clinical work confirms that even in an urban hospital with a large indigent population, most young trauma patients are nutritionally intact at the time of their injury (38). However, standard nutritional indices developed for the elective surgical patient are unreliable in the early postinjury period. The obligatory weight gain due to sodium retention following hemorrhagic shock renders anthropometric measurements virtually uninterpretable. Visceral protein markers, reflected by serum transport protein levels, are likewise distorted by fluid shifts (39) as well as the reprioritization of hepatic protein synthesis (40,41). Albumin, as a constitutive protein, is reduced in the stress period and is shifted out of the intravascular space following hemorrhagic shock (42). Our studies have shown that early postinjury depression in serum albumin most specifically correlates with acute blood loss (43). The sensitivity of these transport proteins also relates to their body pool size and half-life. Prealbumin and retinol-binding protein levels reflect nitrogen deprivation more acutely than serum albumin or transferrin levels, because of the former's relatively small body pool size and short half-life. On the other hand, the unique sensitivity of these rapid-

TABLE 8-1. Nutritional–Immunologic Assessment Used at Denver General Hospital

Routine	Advanced
I. Somatic protein and fat stores 　Height/weight 　Triceps skinfold thickness (TST) 　Arm muscle circumference (AMC) 　　AMC=MAC−(TST × 0.314) 　Creatinine-height index (CHI)	Forearm grip strength
II. Visceral protein status 　Total protein (g/dl) 　Serum albumin (g/dl) 　Serum transferrin (mg/dl)	Prealbumin (mg/dl) Retinol-binding protein (mg/dl)
III. Immune status 　Delayed cutaneous hypersensitivity 　Skin test antigens　　　Results 　Candida (0.1 ml)　　　0 mm=Anergy 　Mumps (0.1 ml)　　　0–5 mm=Rel.anergy 　Coccidioiden (0.1 ml)　5 mm=Normal 　Tuberculin (0.1 ml) 　Total lymphocyte count (mm^3): 　$TLC = \dfrac{WBC \times \% \text{ lymphocytes}}{100}$	Lymphocyte subsets 　(TH:TS ratios) Mitogen-stiumulated 　lymphoproliferation Interleukin production 　(IL-1, IL-2) Granulocyte stem cell 　production Plasma fibronectin 　(μg/dl)
IV. Protein–calorie requirements 　Nitrogen balance 　　Nitrogen in = protein (g) ÷ 6.25 　　Nitrogen out = UUN$_2$ + 3 g 　Resting energy expenditure (HBE) 　　REE (M) = 66 + (13.7W) + (5H) − (6.8A) 　　REE (F) = 655+ (9.6W) +(1.9H) − (4.7A)	Amino acid profile Urinary 3-methylhistadine Indirect calorimetry 　(REE, RQ)

turnover transport proteins compromises their specificity. Cell-mediated immunity, as quantitated by delayed hypersensitivity skin testing, has been embraced as a simple technique to ascertain the impact of malnutrition on host defense (44). In the acute postinjury period, however, tissue disruption, acute hemorrhage, hypovolemic shock, anesthesia, and surgery all significantly depress immune function.

Our interest in nutritional assessment following injury has focused on the decision of which patient who has undergone major abdominal trauma warrants

TABLE 8-2. Abdominal Trauma Index

Organ Injured	Classification
Pancreas	5
Colon	5
Major vascular	5
Duodenum	4
Liver	4
Pelvic fracture	3
Spleen	3
Stomach	3
Kidney	2
Ureter	2
Small bowel	1
Bladder	1
Bone (excluding pelvis)	1
Minor vascular and soft tissue	1
Diaphragm	1
Extrahepatic biliary	1

early aggressive nutritional support. Owing to the inaccuracy of conventional nutritional indices representing physiological and biological markers as outlined above, we utilize the abdominal trauma index (ATI) (45). The ATI is based on anatomical grading and weighing of intra-abdominal injuries, and is calculated at laparotomy (Table 8-2). A severity-of-injury estimate (rated on a scale of 1–5) is assigned to each organ system involved and multiplied by a predetermined risk factor (1–5) for that system. The product of the individual organ scores (risk × severity) produces the total ATI score.

Stress can be estimated clinically by indirect calorimetry. With the advent of the mobile metabolic cart it is feasible to measure respiratory gas exchange to determine carbon dioxide production (VCO_2) and oxygen consumption (VO_2) at the bedside (46). Although the various metabolic carts differ in their specific instrumentation, their operation is fundamentally the same. The concentrations of inspired and expired oxygen (FIO_2 and FEO_2) and concentrations of inspired and expired carbon dioxide (FIO_2 and $FECO_2$) and the expired minute ventilation and accurately measured by open circuit techniques. Interpretation of this data, however, requires knowledge of the patient's condition at study time. Daily nursing care activities or patient agitation produce transient elevations in the Resting Energy Expenditure. Carbon dioxide, unlike oxygen, is stored within the body. This equilibrium is readily disturbed by changes in acid–base status, body temperature, patient activity, and ventilatory pattern. Frequent measurements over several hours are necessary to select steady-state numbers. Mechanical ventilation in itself has pitfalls that have an impact on the interpretation of indirect calorimetry. The FIO_2 must be stable; variations as small as 0.5% result in large errors in calculation. Fluctuations in FIO_2 may also occur with changes in the pressure of the O_2 line source, an unstable internal air–O_2 blender of a ventilator, or mixing of inspired and expired gases. At higher values of FIO_2, analytic determination of the difference between the FIO_2 and FEO_2 creates a greater percentage of error (47). Exhaled tidal volume must be measured accurately. Leaks because of a deflated endotracheal cuff, bronchopleural fistula, or other problems within the system grossly distort this volume. Thus, good understanding of both the metabolic cart and the ventilator is essential to obtain meaningful data.

RATIONALE FOR EARLY NUTRITIONAL SUPPORT

Cofactor of Multiple Organ Failure

Timing of nutritional support in the severely injured but previously well-nourished patient is critical. The postinjury metabolic stress response peaks at 3–4 days and, if not driven by another insult, subsides by day 7–10. The immutable associated hypercatabolism, however, can produce significant protein malnutrition. Accelerated protein turnover permits a limited protein pool to be used efficiently, but when exogenous amino acid supply is insufficient, these amino acids must be derived from endogenous sources (48). Skeletal muscle is the first reserve; when the demand for endogenous amino acids continues, more crucial protein pools are depleted, including visceral structure elements and circulating proteins. Animal studies and clinical observation document that acute protein malnutrition is associated with cardiac, pulmonary, hepatic, gastrointestinal, and immunologic dysfunction (40,50). In essence, a subclinical multiple organ failure syndrome evolves, rendering the patient at greater risk for overwhelming infection.

Multiple organ failure (MOF) is conceptually uncontrolled systemic inflammation resulting in a regional imbalance between supply and demand in life-sustaining systems. Postinjury hypermetabolism is the fundamental background that primes the host for a second or third physiological insult that precipitates the sequential failure of organ systems. Comorbid factors for postinjury MOF are direct organ injury; e.g., pulmonary contusion, major hepatic resection, or pre-existing disease; e.g., hepatic cirrhosis, ischemic heart disease, or chronic pulmonary dysfunction. In 1976, Border (48) suggested that acute protein malnutrition is another insidious risk factor for MOF: when the amino acid oxidative demands cannot be met by skeletal muscle proteolysis. Thus, it is conceivable that failure to provide adequate nutritional support in the first 3–5 days following major trauma may predispose the patient to MOF. This concept has been supported by recent experimental work (51–55) and clinical evidence is beginning to emerge (56).

Clinical Validation: Early Nutrition

Traditional practice has been to delay nutritional support for 5–7 days in the previously well-nourished injured patient, and then TPN is initiated if the individual is unable to consume adequate oral intake. Stimulated by the success of needle catheter jejunostomy (NCJ) following elective gastrointestinal operations reported by Page et al. (57), in 1979 we began a prospective trial to confirm the feasibility of the NCJ in patients sustaining major abdominal trauma (58). Immediate enteral feeding was categorically successful despite extensive injuries, including those of the small bowel and colon. Convinced of the efficacy and safety of the NCJ and prepared with the ATI to identify the high-risk patient, we then conducted a randomized, prospective investigation to analyze the impact of immediate postinjury nutritional support (59). During a 2-1/2 year period, all patients undergoing celiotomy at the Denver General Hospital (DGH) with an abdominal trauma index (ATI) > 15 were entered in a prospective randomized study. Seventy-three (20%) of the 371 injured patients requiring laparotomy during this study period had an ATI > 15. Such patients were randomized to either a control or enteral-fed group. Control patients received conventional D5W (approximately 100 g/day) IV during the first 5 postoperative days, and high-nitrogen TPN (calories/nitrogen = 133:1) by central vein if they were not tolerating a regular diet at that time. The enteral group had an NCJ placed just prior to abdominal closure. Infusion of an elemental diet (Vivonex HN, calories/nitrogen = 150:1) was begun via the jejunal catheter within 12 hrs postoperatively and advanced to meet the metabolic demands within 3 days. Nutritional–immunologic assessment was performed within 12 hr of laparotomy and repeated every third day.

Results of this study are summarized in Table 8-3. The control (n = 31) and enteral-fed (n = 32) groups were comparable with respect to demographic features and injury severity. The groups were also equivalent according to initial nutritional assessment. Twenty (63%) of the 32 enteral-fed patients were maintained on the elemental diet for 5 or more days (range, 5–20; mean, 9 days), while 4 (12%) received TPN. Nine (29%) of the 31 control patients required TPN for a mean duration of 22 days (range, 5–83 days). Significant changes occurred in nitrogen balance at days 4 ($p < 0.025$) and 7 ($p < 0.001$) and in total lymphocyte count at day 7 ($p < 0.05$) in the enteral-fed group. Fifteen (48%) of the 31 control patients developed postoperative complications, and 14 (44%) of the 32 enteral-fed patients did. Although the overall complication rate was similar, septic morbidity was significantly greater ($p < 0.025$) in the control group. Nine

(29%) of the control group developed postoperative infections, consisting of abdominal abscess in seven and major pneumonia in two. This compared with three (9%) of the early-fed group, all of whom developed an abdominal abscess. Moreover, the mean ATI of patients developing complications in the control group was 31, while in the enteral group it was 48. The cost savings exceeded $3,000.00 per patient in the enteral-fed group. Thus, this prospective randomized study demonstrated a statistically significant reduction in septic morbidity following major abdominal trauma as a result of nutritional support immediately post-injury.

Route of Delivery: TEN vs. TPN

Once one has acknowledged the benefit of early nutrition in the high-risk patient, the next question is the preferred route of substrate delivery: total enteral nutrition (TEN) or TPN. Safety, convenience, and cost are the commonly stated advantages of enteral nutrition (60). The gut has been inappropriately perceived as a dormant organ following stress. Nasogastric decompression is typically required for 1–2 days postinjury due to loss of gastric motility, while colon peristalsis is impaired for 3–5 days; but small-bowel motility and absorption remain functionally intact despite laparotomy or acute stress. With the advent of nasojejunal tubes and the NCJ to allow access to the small bowel, plus refinement to enteral diets, immediate postoperative jejunal feeding has been shown to be simple, safe, and effective in a wide variety of surgical patients (61–64).

The injury stress response is the net result of both macroendocrine (the classic stress hormones) and microendocrine (inflammatory mediators) stimuli and prolonged stress sets the stage for progressive multiple organ failure. The preservation of intestinal mucosa and limited portal and systemic bacterial endotoxemia are therefore paramount. The gut provides an essential barrier to enteric flora and their endotoxins (65). Several investigators have proved convincingly that bacteria migrate: "bacterial translocation" from the intestinal lumen into regional lymph nodes, liver, spleen as well as into existing abdominal abscesses (66–68). Bacterial translocation from the gut to the liver has been shown to suppress systemic T-cell-mediated immunity, possibly by augmenting production of prostaglandins from Kupffer's cells (69). Macrophage-induced modulation of liver protein synthesis may also occur due to release of interleukin-1, a known trigger for hepatic acute phase protein synthesis, tumor necrosis factor, or other mediators (70). Gastrointestinal atrophy is a well-defined phenomenon in humans as well as animals fed exclusively by vein. There is marked atrophy of the stomach, duodenum, jejunum, and pancreas in otherwise well-nourished subjects maintained on TPN (71). More recent work has confirmed reduced villous height and suppressed crypt cell proliferation in the inactive small bowel (72). Other investigators have confirmed substantial changes in systemic levels of gut-derived hormones: gastrin, glucagon, insulin, gastric inhibitory peptide, and vasoactive intestinal peptide, associated with TPN (72,73).

During stress, net skeletal muscle proteolysis releases large quantities of alanine and glutamine. There is accelerated uptake of glutamine by the gastrointestinal tract, and circulating as well as tissue glutamine levels are depressed. The gut adapts to spare glucose for obligate users; glutamine becomes the preferred metabolic fuel of the gastrointestinal mucosa (30). Standard TPN does not contain glutamine and this may contribute to the impaired enterocyte function observed during critical illness. Indeed, recent studies with glutamine-enriched TPN have demonstrated an attenuation of TPN-associated gut atrophy. In other studies, the addition of epidermal growth factor has also been effective in maintaining gut mucosal integrity (72–74). Comparative animal studies have shown that TEN improves resistance to experimental peritonitis and enhances biliary production of secretory IgA (52–54). Early enteral alimentation also appears to blunt the hypercatabolism associated with thermal injury. Alexander et al. (55,56) demonstrated that enterally fed animals had greater jejunal mucosal weight and thickness, more normal resting metabolic expenditure, and lower glucagon and cortisol levels when feedings were begun at 2 hr vs. 72 hr postburn. Taken together, these animals data suggest that early enteral alimentation decreases bacterial translocation from the gut lumen, reduces the postinjury hypercatabolic state, and improves host resistance to infection.

There is a paucity of well-controlled randomized, prospective studies comparing TEN to TPN in the critically injured patient. Our clinical study in patients with major abdominal trauma, demonstrating a significant reduction in septic complications as a result of immediate TEN, prompted a subsequent study designed to ascertain whether early TPN would produce equivalent benefits (75). Fifty patients with an ATI >15 and <40 were randomized at initial laparotomy to receive either TEN (Vivonex TEN) or TPN (Freamine HBC 6.9% and Trophamine 6%); both regimens contained 2.5% fat, 33% branched-chain amino acids, and had a calorie/nitrogen ratio of 150:1. Nutritional support was initiated within 12 hr postoperatively in both groups, and infused at a rate sufficient to render the patients in positive nitrogen balance within 48 hr. TEN was delivered via a needle catheter jejunostomy by a protocol described in the next section. The study groups (TEN 29 vs. TPN 30) were comparable in age (28.3 ± 1.9 vs. 31.4 ± 2.4 years), injury severity (ATI = 24.7 ± 1.1 vs 24.0 ± 1.0; injury severity score = 28.7 ± 2.3 vs. 25.1 ± 1.0), and initial metabolic stress (day 1 urine urea nitrogen [UUN_2] = 8.6 ± 0.8 vs. 9.4 ± 0.9 g; day 1 REE = 1641 ± 42 vs 1731 ± 58 kCal). Jejunal feeding was tolerated unconditionally in 25 (86%) of the TEN patients. Three patients required manipulations in the feeding schedule, while the remaining patient required a transitional period with supplemental TPN. The TPN group received slightly more protein and calories, but

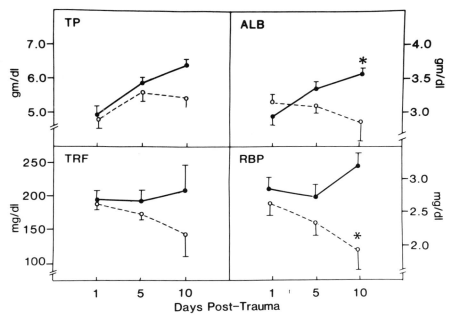

Figure 8-1. Traditional nutritional indices include total protein (TP), albumin (ALB), transferrin (TRF), and retinal binding protein (RBP). Mean SEM is shown at days 1, 5, and 10. Statistically significant differences (ALB, $p = 0.004$; RBP, $p = 0.02$) between groups are marked with an asterisk. Total enteral nutrition (TEN) is denoted by a solid line (———) and total parental nutrition (TPN) is denoted by a dotted line (- - - - -).

nitrogen balance remained equivalent throughout the study period (day 5 TEN = 0.3 ± 1.0; TPN = 0.1 ± 0.8 g/day). Significant differences occurred in the levels of standard visceral protein markers over time (Figure 8-1). Total protein, albumin, transferrin, and retinol-binding protein levels all increased over the study period in the TEN group, while they decreased in the TPN patients.

To test the hypothesis that enteral nutrition reduces bacterial translocation, we examined reprioritization of hepatic protein synthesis. Reprioritization was defined as the relative balance of acute-phase proteins compared to constitutive proteins (nonacute phase). Specific serum protein levels were profiled using crossed immunoelectrophoresis. Prealbumin and α2-macroglobulin (α2-M) were considered representative of constitutive protein synthesis, while haptoglobin, orosomucord, and α1-antitrypsin (α1-AT) were chosen to reflect acute-phase protein synthesis. Figure 8-2 shows typical posttraumatic hepatic protein synthesis reprioritization when the TEN and TPN groups were combined. The level of haptoglobin, an acute-phase protein, increased threefold by 5 days and then

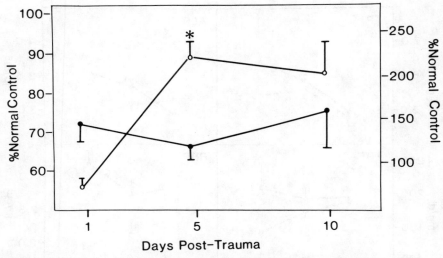

Figure 8-2. Percent normal control (mean and SEM) for groups receiving enteral nutrition and total parenteral nutrition was combined at days 1, 5, and 10. The statistically significant difference ($p = 0.0001$) from the baseline is marked with an asterisk. Prealbumin is denoted by a solid line (――――) and heptoglobin is denoted by a dotted line (- - - - -).

returned to normal. In contrast, the level of prealbumin, a non-acute-phase protein, decreased at day 5 and then returned to normal. When these results are segregated by treatment groups, divergent patterns of protein synthesis emerged. Figure 8-3A shows that $\alpha 2$-M levels are equally depressed in the TPN and TEN groups at day 1; by day 5, levels had risen slightly. On day 10, however, the $\alpha 2$-M level in the TEN group had returned to normal levels while remaining depressed in the TPN group. When analyzed from another perspective, Figure 8-3B shows that the difference for TEN and TPN groups (an increase in baseline to day 10 for $\alpha 2$-M) was significantly greater for the TEN patients. Similar trends were seen for prealbumin. In contrast, levels of the serum acute-phase protein $\alpha 1$-AT increased to a greater degree in the TPN group than in the TEN group. Baseline levels were similar for both groups. At day 5, however, $\alpha 1$-AT levels in the TPN group increased more than in the TEN group. Levels in both treatment groups fell slightly by day 10. These data suggest that TEN ameliorates reprioritization of hepatic protein synthesis following major torso trauma. Although these results are speculative, we believe that this reflects a reduction in bacterial translocation by preservation of gut mucosal integrity. The clinical impact of these findings was collaborated by a significant difference in septic morbidity between the groups. Five (17%) of the TEN patients compared to 11 (37%) of the TPN group ($p < 0.02$) developed postoperative infections. Moreover, the

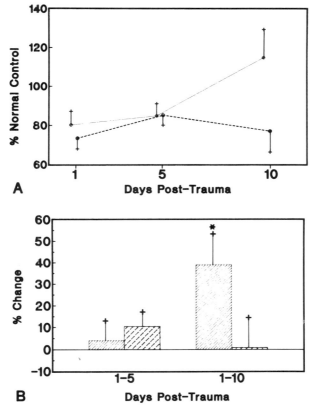

Figure 8-3. α_2—MacroglobulinPercent normal control (mean and SEM) is shown at days 1, 5, and 10. The statistically significant difference (p = 0.04) between groups is marked with an asterisk. Total enteral nutrition (TEN) is denoted by a solid line (————) and total parental nutrition (TPN) is denoted by a dotted line (- - - - -).

incidence of major septic morbidity was 3% (one abdominal abscess) in the TEN group in contrast to 20% (two abdominal abscess, four pneumonia) with TPN.

PROTOCOL FOR POSTINJURY NUTRITIONAL SUPPORT

Early Enteral Feeding

Our proposed nutritional support for major abdominal trauma is summarized in Figure 8-4. Patients with an ATI >15, or the equivalent using another injury

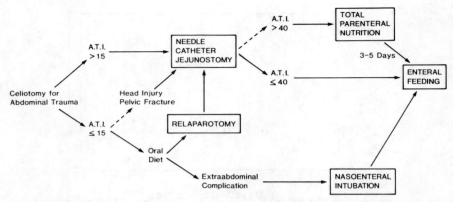

Figure 8-4. Proposed nutritional support plan for patients sustaining acute major abdominal trauma based on the intraoperative abdominal trauma index (ATI).

severity index, have an NCJ placed at emergency laparotomy unless re-exploration is planned within 48 hr. In the latter situation the catheter is placed more safely at the second operation. The NCJ is also warranted for patients with an ATI < 15 in whom associated extra-abdominal injuries (e.g., severe head injury or major pelvic crush) will prolong their catabolic state. However, in these patients, as well as in patients with extensive intra-abdominal injury (ATI > 40) or massive blood loss (> 25 units) in which reflex small bowel ileus is likely (76), TPN is initiated with transition to jejunostomy feeding within 3–5 days. The NCJ is also placed in patients undergoing reoperation for presumed abdominal infections; sepsis does not preclude jejunal feeding in this clinical setting (77).

Placement of Needle Catheter Jejunostomy

Our technique for NCJ (Figure 8-5) is similar to that described originally by Delany and associates (78). An NCJ kit is available commercially (Norwich Eaton Pharmaceutical) and consists of a 90 cm 5 F radiopaque polyurethane feeding catheter; a 100-cm, Teflon-coated, flexible stainless steel stylet; two 14-gauge, 5-cm, thin-walled needles; an 18-gauge blunt adapter needle; and an 8 Fr polyurethane catheter sleeve retainer. The NCJ is placed at the completion of the operative procedure, just before the abdominal cavity is closed. The site for insertion is the most proximal small bowel that will reach the anterior or lateral abdominal wall without tension, usually 15 cm beyond the ligament of Trietz or an equivalent distance from the anastomosis in the efferent loop of a Roux-en-Y jejunostomy or gastrojejunostomy. A purse-string seromuscular suture of 3-0 silk is placed in the antimesenteric border of the jejunum at the entrance site. A submucosal tunnel is created in the jejunal wall with a 14-gauge, 5-cm needle. This prevents reflux around the catheter during feeding and allows

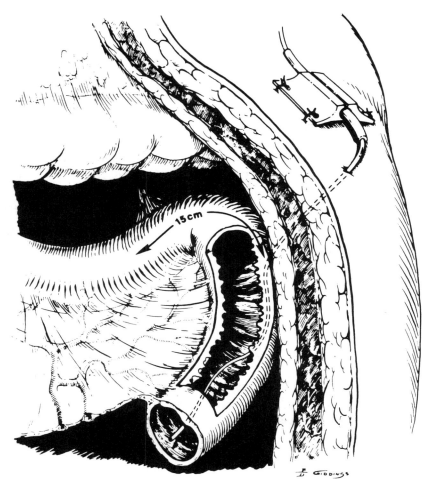

Figure 8-5. A needle catheter jejunostomy is placed at initial laparotomy in patients with an abdominal trauma index (ATI) of greater than 15.

for closure of the jejunal wall when the catheter is removed. The tunnel is created by introducing the needle, with the bevel point up, through the purse-string suture. The needle is advanced its full length in the submucosal layer of the bowel, and then rotated 180 degrees as the needle is introduced into the bowel lumen. The flexible tip of the stylet is identified, and this end of the catheter is passed through the 14-gauge needle into the bowel lumen. The needle is then extracted, the catheter advanced approximately 25 cm, and the stylet removed by gentle traction. The 3-0 silk purse-string suture is tied to seal the submucosal tunnel at the serosal level of the jejunum. The suture should not be wrapped around the catheter because this will hamper removal. An exit site for the catheter is chosen on the abdominal wall where the loop of jejunum containing the catheter can reach without tension. A second 14-gauge, 5-cm needle is then passed through this point from the skin surface into the peritoneal cavity. This needle should be introduced at a slight angle paralleling the axis of the catheter as it exits the gut. The catheter is then threaded retrograde through this needle to exit the abdominal wall. The loop of jejunum is fixed to the abdominal wall with two 3-0 polyglycolic acid sutures, placed 2 cm cephalad and 2 cm caudad to the catheter entrance site. These sutures should be placed to ensure a gradual curve in the transfixed loop of bowel to avoid a point fixation about which the gut may rotate. The extra-abdominal segment of catheter is shortened to 10 cm, and a blunt 18-gauge needle inserted. The catheter is then anchored to the skin. Finally, a 10 ml bolus of normal saline solution is injected through the catheter to confirm free flow. The most common cause of resistance is kinking due to a tight suture; this must be corrected before the abdomen is closed.

Postoperative Management and GI Tolerance

We currently prefer an elemental diet for our injured patients, enriched with branched-chain amino acids BCAA and low in viscosity to facilitate infusion via small-bore catheter. A relatively normal pH as well as low fat content in the diet are important to limit biliopancreatic stimulation (79). Our clinical experience to date has demonstrated the safety of an elemental diet in patients with pancreatic as well as distal intestinal injury. We start jejunostomy feedings within 12 hr postinjury, beginning the elemental diet at a concentration of 0.25 kCal/ml. The solution is infused at a constant rate, using an enteral infusion pump, and increased in volume, then in concentration, at 8-hr intervals until 125–150 ml/hr of three-quarter-strength solution is delivered (Table 8-3). The total calories are individualized according to the patient's energy requirements for effective nitrogen utilization, corroborated by indirect calorimetry. In the early postinjury period following multiple intestinal perforations, gastric decompression is important to avert the rare occurrence of pneumatosis intestinalis (80).

Despite the increasing evidence for early feeding, there is reluctance among surgeons to begin enteral nutrition immediately postinjury due to alleged intolerance by patients. We recently reviewed 130 patients requiring emergency laparotomy for major abdominal trauma (ATI $>$ 15) who had been randomized in sequential studies to receive TPN or TEN (63). The enteral diet was administered by the previously outlined protocol, nasogastric decompression maintained for at least 48 hr, and no patient received supplemental albumin. On daily questioning, 50% of the TPN group noted gastrointestinal (GI) complaints, 13% were graded moderate or severe; 83% of the TEN patients experienced GI distress.

TABLE 8-3. Clinical Benefits of Early Postinjury Nutritional Support

Study Day	Albumin (mg/dl)	Transferrin (mg/dl)	Total Lymphocyte Count (cell/mm^3)	N$_2$ Balance (g/day)	Sepsis	Cost/ Patient
Control (n = 13)						
1	3.3±0.1	223±7	1,408±158	−13.2±0.5	9	$19,636
4	3.1±0.1	187±5	1,175±176	−11.4±0.7	(29%)	
7	3.3±0.1	213±9	1,482±138	−11.1±0.7		
Enteral (n = 32)						
1	3.3±0.1	223±6	1,831±206	−13.7±0.7	3[a]	
4	3.2±0.1	184±7	1,344±166	−3.9±1.6	(9%)	$16,280
7	3.2±0.1	211±10	2,054±164*	−5.2±1.3		

Values are given as ± standard error of mean (SEM).
[a]$P \leq 0.05$.

When graded, 35% of the enteral fed patients had moderate or severe symptoms, 15% required adjustment of the feeding schedule, and 13% had their protocol changed to TPN. This clinical experience indicates that most patients sustaining major abdominal trauma have postoperative GI complaints, but these complaints do not preclude aggressive enteral feeding. With attentive management by an experienced team, 90% of these patients will tolerate full-scale enteral feeding. The 13% intolerance rate is usually associated with extensive abdominal injury (ATI > 40), major pelvic fractures (grade III vertical shear or anteroposterior compression), or massive intraoperative blood transfusion requirements (> 25 units).

Abdominal cramping and secondary distention usually occur at the initiation of the diet and are minimized by progressing the feedings in a gradual fashion. If these complaints develop, the infusion is regressed one step on the administration schedule for an additional 8 hr (Table 8-4). Nasogastric output should be monitored in such patients and the enteral diet colored with methylene blue to exclude reflux into the stomach. If cramping and distention do not resolve despite adjustments in feeding, the enteral infusion should be temporarily discontinued and the patient evaluated for ileus, intestinal obstruction, or pneumatosis intestinalis. An abdominal plain roentgenogram is helpful. Persistent diarrhea is uncommon with enteral feeding in our experience and is usually controlled by slowing the rate of administration. In refractory cases, paragoric may be added to the solution, beginning with 10 mg/L, not to exceed a maximum concentration of 30 mg/L.

Technical complications resulting from NCJ are rare. Resistance to gravity infusion in the immediate postoperative period is usually due to a constricting

TABLE 8-4. Administration Schedule for Jejunostomy Feeding in Patient with Abdominal Trauma

0.25 kcal/ml @ 50 ml/hr × 8 hours
0.25 kcal/ml @ 75 ml/hr × 8 hours
0.25 kcal/ml @ 100 ml/hr × 8 hours
0.50 kcal/ml @ 100 ml/hr × 8 hours
0.75 kcal/ml @ 100 ml/hr × 8 hours
1.00 kcal/ml @ 100 ml/hr × 8 hours
1.00 kcal/ml @ 125 ml/hr[a]

[a]If caloric requirements warrant.

suture, which is easily remedied if at the skin level but problematic if within the abdominal cavity. In the latter situation, withdrawing the catheter several centimeters may resolve the problem. Delayed catheter occlusion is usually due to accumulation of debris within the catheter. The problem may be ameliorated by flushing the catheter with hydrogen peroxide. If there is inadvertent catheter dislodgement, a contrast study should be obtained to verify the final resting position of the intra-abdominal catheter.

The enteral solution is mixed in a large-capacity blender and stored in clean plastic containers under refrigeration. After 48 hr, unused diet is discarded. Only enough solution to infuse over 8 hr is kept at the patient's bedside. Washing the blender by hand after every mixing, rinsing the administration set between feedings, and changing the set daily will also reduce bacterial proliferation in the diet (81,82). One of the major virtues of enteral feeding is the paucity of fluid, electrolyte, and metabolic complications, although the array of complications common with TPN can occur with TEN. Our practice is to infuse enteral solution continuously at an appropriate rate until the patient is able to tolerate adequate oral intake. If the recuperating patient appears to have a suppressed appetite, we will convert to cyclic feeding: i.e., supplemental nutrition during the night only.

Total Parenteral Nutrition

Total parenteral nutrition is used in patients requiring nutritional support in whom enteral feeding is impractical or unsuccessful. A specific problematic group of patients are those who have sustained massive abdominal injury with an ATI > 40 (see Figure 8-4). In this group we initiate TPN with transition to enteral feedings in 3–5 days as tolerated. In patients in whom enteral feeding must be terminated because of intraperitoneal sepsis that requires reoperation, TPN is used for support until the GI tract has recovered sufficiently to absorb the enteral diet.

Parenteral solutions with an osmolarity exceeding 800 mOsm/L generally thrombose peripheral veins and thus mandate infusion via central vein. Various techniques of central venous cannulation are described well in other reviews (83); we prefer the infraclavicular subclavian (84) or posterior internal jugular vein approaches (85). Our standard central venous catheter policy includes strict aseptic techniques for all catheter manipulations and dressing changes. Central venous catheters are changed routinely over a wire every 5 days and the tip sent for semiquantitative culture. If catheter sepsis is suspected, the site is changed. Criteria for catheter sepsis include a site with purulent drainage, the same organism identified on the catheter tip and blood cultures, two sequential positive catheter tip cultures, or two positive blood cultures without an obvious source in conjunction with pain and erythema at the catheter site. The sterile transparent dressings are changed every other day by the staff nurse. A 24-hr supply of TPN is mixed under sterile conditions in the hospital pharmacy. This complete nutritive admixture is administered in a 3 L bag delivery system that is changed daily (86). A Luer-Lok connector is used to connect the administration set to the central catheter; no filters are included in the TPN administration equipment. Continuing monitoring of this protocol has demonstrated a catheter infection rate consistently below 3.5%.

Selecting the appropriate TPN formula is another controversial issue. The regimens we currently use are outlined in Table 8-5. The primary differences include type of caloric source, amino acid composition, and nonprotein calorie/nitrogen ratio. Each TPN formula is supplemented with a standard profile of essential vitamins and minerals, unless specific deficiencies are identified. Additional electrolyte or insulin requirements are adjusted as needed; otherwise, they are provided via separate peripheral intravenous (IV) line. Vitamin K and iron (Imferon) are administered by intramuscular (IM) injection. Although the individual selection of nutritional formulas is somewhat arbitrary, we rely on the stress regimen as the mainstay in our severely injured patients. This formula is designed to have a low calorie/nitrogen ratio and an elevated branched-chain amino acid content that increases the total nitrogen load. Approximately 22% of the calories is given as lipid (0.5–1.0 g/kg) and the rest as dextrose. We convert to the mixed-fuel formula, providing a more balanced provision of calories when the patient's acute hypermetabolic state has subsided, usually assessed by nitrogen balance studies or the metabolic cart. The carbohydrate solution is generally reserved for patients in whom lipid clearance is a problem, as reflected by persistent elevated plasma triglyceride levels (87). In patients with established multiple organ failure in whom dialysis is required, we use the stress formula and determine nitrogen demands by the Sargent equation for urea nitrogen generation (88,89).

Enthusiasm for peripheral TPN has vacillated considerably over the past decade. The advent of safe lipid emulsions has facilitated nutritional support via the peripheral route, but the potential immunologic penalty has reopened the

TABLE 8-5. Adult Total Parenteral Nutrition Formulas (Denver General Hospital)

	Postinjury Stress Formula	Recovery Mixed Fuel Formula	Recovery Carbohydrate-Base	Recovery Peripheral
Protein (%)	4.5% amino acids (45% BCAA)	4.1% amino acids	4.25% amino acids	2.4 amino acids
Nitrogen (gm/L)	6.5 gm/L	6.5 g/L	6.8 g/L	3.7 g/L
Nonprotein (kcal/L)	743 kcal/L	1000 kcal/L	850 kcal/L	504 kcal/L
% Lipid (g)	22% (18 g/L)	40% (23 g/L)	−(100 g biweekly)	79% (40g/L)
% Dextrose (g)	78% (168 g/L)	60% (182 g/L)	100% (250 g/L)	21% (24 g glycerol)
Nonprotein Kcal/N_2 ratio	113:1	153:1	125:1	137:1

TPN formula is supplemented with:

Electrolytes/minerals (per L)	*Vitamins (per day)*	*Trace elements (per day)*	*Vitamin K*
Sodium 25 mEq	Ascorbic acid 100mg	Zinc 3.0mg	4mg IM/Week
Potassium 33 mEq	Vitamin A 3,00 IU	Copper 1.2mg	Imferon 0.5mg
Phosphate 13 mEq	Vitamin D 200 IU	Manganese 0.3mg	IM/Week
Calcium 5 mEq	Thiamine HCI 3mg	Chromium 12ug	
Magnesium 5 mEq	Riboflavin 3.6mg		
Acjetate 25 mEq	Pyridoxin 4mg		
Chloride 25 mEq	Niacinamide 40mg		
	Dexpantheral 15mg		
	Biotin 60ug		
	Folic acid 400ug		
	Vitamin B_{12} 5ug		

question of safety (90). Most recently, glycerol has been added to the regimen and appears to be an effective nitrogen-sparing substrate (91). Despite these advances, peripheral TPN is usually inadequate to support the severely catabolic patient. In general, we use the peripheral TPN formula in patients who are reasonably well nourished, moderately stressed, and in whom we anticipate oral feeding within 1 week.

CASE STUDY

A 23-year-old worker fell 25 feet onto a concrete floor of a warehouse, landing on his right side. When paramedics arrived, he was in profound shock and transported immediately to the Emergency Department. On arrival, the patient had a pulse of 120/min and a systolic blood pressure of less than 80 mmHg. Initial evaluation revealed fractures of the right posterior ribs 8–11 and transverse process fractures of L1–L5. His urine was grossly bloody, and his diagnostic peritoneal lavage yielded copious free blood. Due to continued hypovolemic hemorrhagic shock, the patient was oral–tracheally intubated, infused with type-specific blood, and taken promptly to the operating room. A broad-spectrum antibiotic was administered in the Emergency Department.

A midline abdominal incision revealed a massive injury to the right lobe of the liver with obvious involvement of the retrohepatic vena cava (grade V injury). A Pringle maneuver was performed, the liver packed tightly, and further stabilization efforts continued. The interior vena cava was repaired using a balloon shunt, but the patient's course was complicated by profound metabolic acidosis, (initial pH, 5.5), core hypothermia (30–32°C), and persistent shock. Efforts to reverse his hypothermia and hypoxemia were ultimately successful using a combination of resuscitative maneuvers including blood warmers, heated ventilation, and closed chest lavage using preheated crystalloid, but a profound coagulopathy ensued. Approximately 2 hr postinjury, his prothrombin time (PT) and partial thrombopeastin time (PTT) were markedly prolonged, and platelet count was less than 12,000/mm^3, despite transfusion of more than 63 units of whole blood products. Liver packing was not successful in controlling hemorrhage and a Longmire clamp was placed across the right hepatic lobe to control the recalcitrant bleeding. The abdomen was closed with towel clips to expedite transfer of the patient to the intensive care unit.

While in the ICU the patient received an additional 17 units of whole blood and 50 units of blood components. He was returned to the operating room 16 hr later without clinical evidence of active bleeding or coagulopathy. During his abdominal re-exploration, careful removal of the packing and clots produced little new bleeding and a right hepatic lobectomy was completed at the margin of the Longmire clamp. The patient also had a tracheostomy placed for postoperative respiratory care and a decompressive gastrostomy as well as a needle catheter jejunostomy placed for postoperative enteral feeding.

Stress TPN was begun initially, with the rate advanced over 8 hr to provide 2200 nonprotein kCal and 18 g N$_2$ (2 g Pro/Kg) per day (see Table 8-6). Despite the early development of acute renal failure and hepatic dysfunction, an aggressive regime of elevated branched-chain amino acids, low fat and low kCal/N$_2$ ratio TPN was continued as attempts at enteral feeding were begun. The NCJ feeding was initially delayed due to the severity of his liver injury and massive blood transfusion, but on day 4 postinjury the enteral diet was begun at a low volume and dilute concentration. Over the next 2 days the TPN was gradually weaned and the enteral diet advanced, with a transition to full enteral nutrition by day 8 postinjury. Over the next 3 days, the acute respiratory distress syndrome

TABLE 8-6. Nutritional Profile of 23-Year-Old Victim of Blunt Trauma

	Postoperative Day				
	1	7	12	18	22
Weight (kg)	81	70	71	71	67
Total protein (gm/dL)	4.8	5.1	5.0	6.6	6.6
Albumin (g/DL)	2.6	2.5	2.3	2.8	2.9
Transferrin	144	132	109	136	223
Total lymphocyte count cells/mm^3	2,800	1,360	1,200	1,700	1,200
SGOT (U/L)	101	152	117	191	119
Alkaline phosphatase (U/L)	113	90	242	341	394
Total bilirubin (mg/dL)	23	10.3	2.8	3.4	3.2
Serum creatine (mg/dL)	1.7	1.5	1.1	0.9	1.1
Urine urea N$_2$ (gm/day)	11.4	16.3	18.6	11.4	—
N$_2$ balance	+2.9	+1.2	1.7	+3.2	—
REE kilocalories/24 hr	2,133	2,270	2,077	—	—
RQ	1.14	1.04	1.12	—	—

(ARDS) as well as the renal and liver dysfunction resolved. However, on day 11 postinjury, the patient developed a hemodynamic profile suggestive of sepsis. He was nevertheless maintained on full enteral nutrition. Surveillance cultures disclosed *Candida* in the urine and blood, and a course of amphotericin eradicated his infection, allowing him to be weaned from mechanical ventilation. Once free of the ventilator and capable of good swallowing mechanics, the patient was advanced to a soft diet and the NCJ feedings were discontinued. The patient was discharged 47 days postinjury after full rehabilitation.

FUTURE CONSIDERATIONS

Tremendous progress has been achieved in nutritional support over the past two decades. However, in the year 2000 the 1990s will probably be viewed as a transition period from nearly exclusive TPN to a balance with TEN. The primary impetus has been recognition of the potential role the gut plays in the pathogenesis of multiple organ failure. There remains much to learn about the complex metabolic, immunologic, and bacteriologic regulatory functions of the gastrointestinal tract, and how they are altered by acute stress (92,93). The strong interdependence of the gut and other organs is now being appreciated.

There are an endless number of highly controversial clinical issues concerning nutritional support practices: optimal nutrients for the critically ill patient, e.g., branched-chain amino acids (leucine), specific amino acids (glutamine, arginine), fatty acids (n-3, n-6), minerals (zinc), vitamins (A,C) etc.; the relative balance of substrate, e.g., calorie/nitrogen ratio, fat/carbohydrate, peptides vs. amino acids, and so on; tailoring nutrients for the patient with pulmonary, hepatic, or renal failure. One of the major clinical research challenges will be to validate in humans the basic pathophysiological and metabolic concepts demonstrated by animal investigations (94). Our current clinical research focus is a prospective, randomized comparative study of Immun-Aid (McGaw, Inc.) a new enteral diet with immune-enhancing characteristics, and Vivonex TEN in patients with abdominal trauma. Supplemented with glutamine, arginine, n-3 fatty acids, and nucleic acids, Immun-Aid is designed to provide tissue-specific nutrients that not only enhance gut mucosal integrity but also modulate monocyte/lymphocyte function to reverse postoperative immunosuppression.

Clinical confirmation of improved gut preservation (74,94) and enhanced nitrogen retention (95) with glutamine-enriched TPN has significant implications, particularly in the management of the patient who cannot be fed enterally. Another area that appears promising is the addition of growth factors with TPN to restore gastrointestinal integrity (96,97). A variety of peptide growth factors (GF) (epidermal GF, transforming GF-B, fibroblast GF, platelet-derived GF, etc.) have been shown to stimulate cellular proliferation by autocrine or paracrine activity. Epidermal GF has been shown to have trophic effects on small bowel mucosa in animals, which are additive to those achieved by glutamine-enriched TPN. Other studies have shown that both systemic and luminal epidermal GF increase intestinal substrate absorption without changes in mucosa DNA levels. It is assumed that the gut releases growth factors that have local effects on intestinal epithelium as well as a direct impact on the liver via the portal vein and distant organs through the lymphatic circulation. Thus, while the current focus is on gut-derived endotoxin, other factors released by the gastrointestinal tract may have a more profound influence on the response to injury and ultimate risk of lethal multiple organ failure.

REFERENCES

1. Bliss DW: Feeding per rectum: as illustrated in the case of the late President Garfield and others. Med Rec 22:64–65, 1882.
2. Edsal DL, Miller CW: Study of two cases nourished exclusively per rectum; with a determination of absorption nitrogen metabolism and intestinal putre faction. Trans Coll Physicians 24:225, 1902.
3. Schackelford RT: Surgery of the Alimentary Tract. Philadelphia: W.B. Saunders, 1986.
4. Wolfer JA: Jejunostomy with jejunal alimentation. Ann Surg 101:708, 1935.

5. Torosian MH, Rombeau JL: Feeding by tube enterostomy. Surg Gynecol Obstet 150:918, 1980.
6. Andresen AFR: Immediate jejunal feeding after gastroenterostomy. Ann Surg 67:565, 1918.
7. Abbott WO, Rawson AJ: A tube for use in the postoperative care of gastroenterostomy patients—a correction. JAMA 112:2414, 1939.
8. Moss G, et al: Postoperative metabolic patterns following immediate total nutritional support: hormone levels, DNA synthesis, nitrogen balance and accelerated wound healing. J Surg Res 21:383, 1976.
9. MacDonald AH: Intrajejunal drip in gastric surgery. Lancet 73:786, 1954.
10. Delany HM, et al: Jejunostomy by needle catheter technique. Surgery 73:786, 1973.
11. Page CP, et al: Continued catheter administration of an elemental diet. Surg Gynecol Obstet 142:184, 1976.
12. Fischer JE: Metabolism in surgical patients. Protein, carbohydrate, and fat utilization by oral and parenteral routes. In Sabiston DL (ed) Textbook of Surgery: The Biological Basis of Modern Surgical Practice. Philadelphia: W.B. Saunders, 1986.
13. Philosophical Transactions of the Royal Society of London (1656), abridged copy. London, 45:1809.
14. Lowen R, James R: Transfusion Medicinal Dictionary. London 1745, Volume III, cities Philosophical Transactions for December 17, 1666.
15. Cerra FB: Pocket Manual of Surgical Nutrition. St. Louis: C.V.Mosby, 1984.
16. Henrique V, Anderson AC: Monatsschr Physiol Chem 88:357, 1913.
17. Cuthbertson DP: Further observations on the disturbance of metabolism caused by injury, with particular reference to the dietary requirements of fracture cases. Br J Surg 23:505, 1935.
18. Elman R: Series of patients with improved hydrolysate. Ann Surg 112:594, 1940.
19. Rose WD, et al: Recognition of essential and non-essential amino acids. Phys Rev 18:109, 1939.
20. Rhode CM, et al: Method for continuous intravenous administration of nutritive solutions suitable for prolonged metabolic studies in dogs. Am J Physiol 159:409, 1949.
21. Dudrick SJ, et al: Long term parenteral nutrition with growth, development and positive nitrogen balance. Surgery 64:134, 1968.
22. Bessey PQ, Watters JM, Aoki TT, et al: Combined hormonal infusion stimulates the metabolic response to injury. Ann Surg 200:264, 1984.
23. Bessey PQ, Jiank Z, Johnson DJ, et al: Posttraumatic skeletal muscle proteolysis: The role of the hormonal environment. World J Surg 13:465, 1989.
24. Clowes GHA, Hirsch E, George BC, et al: Survival from sepsis—the significance of altered protein metabolism regulated by proteolysis inducting factor, the circulating cleavage product of interleukin-I. Ann Surg 202:446, 1985.
25. Warren RS, Starnes F, Gabrilove JL, et al: The acute metabolic effects of tumor necrosis factor administration in humans. Arch Surg 122:1396, 1987.

26. Moldawer LL, Svaninger G, Gelin J, et al: Interleukin-1 and tumor necrosis factor do not regulate protein balance in skeletal muscle. Am J Physiol 2553:766, 1987.
27. Birkhahn RH, Long CL, Fitkin D, et al: Effect of major skeletal trauma on whole body protein turnover in man measured by L-(1,^{14}C-)-leucine. Surgery 88:294, 1908.
28. Cerra F, Blackburn G, Hirsch J, et al: The effect of stress level, amino acid formula and nitrogen dose on nitrogen retention in traumatic and septic stress. Ann Surg 205:282, 1987.
29. Sax HC, Talamini MA, Fischer JE: Clinical use of branched-chain acids in liver disease, sepsis, trauma, and burns. Arch Surg 121:348, 1986.
30. Souba WW, Smith RJ, Wilmore DW: Glutamine metabolism by the intestinal tract. JPEN 9:603, 1985.
31. Askanazi J, Carpentier YA, Michelsen CB, et al: Muscle and plasma amino acids following injury. Ann Surg 192:78, 1980.
32. Barbul A: Arginine: biochemistry, physiology, and therapeutic implications. JPEN 10:227, 1986.
33. Black PR, Brooks, DC, Bessey, PQ, et al: Mechanisms of insulin resistance. Ann Surg 196:420, 1982.
34. Birkhahn RH, Long CI, Fitkin DL, et al: A comparison of the effects of skeletal trauma and surgery on the ketosis of starvation in man. J Trauma 21:513, 1981.
35. Harris RL, Frenkel RA, Cotton GL, et al: Lipid mobilization and metabolism after thermal trauma. J Trauma 22:194, 1982.
36. Robin AP, Askanazi J, Greenwood RC, et al: Lipoprotein lipase activity in surgical patients: influence of trauma and infection. Surgery 90:401, 1981.
37. Kolpek JH, Ott LG, Record KE, et al: Comparison of urinary urea nitrogen excretion and measured energy expenditure in spinal cord injury and nonsteroid-treated severe head trauma patients. JPEN 13:277, 1989.
38. Moore EE, Jones, TN: Nutritional assessment and preliminary report on early support of the trauma patient. J Am Coll Nutr 2:45, 1983.
39. Elwyn DH, Bryan-Brown CW, Shoemaker WC: Nutritional aspects of body water dislocation in postoperative and depleted patients. Ann Surg 182:76, 1975.
40. Peterson VM, Moore EE, Jones TN, et al: TEN versus TPN following major torso injury; attenuation of hepatic protein reprioritization. Surgery 104:199, 1988.
41. Shetty PS, Jung RT, Watrasiewicz KE, et al: Rapid turnover transport proteins—an index of subclinical and depleted-energy malnutrition. Lancet 2:230, 1979.
42. Lucas CE, Ledgerwood AM: Reduced oncotic pressure after shock—A proposed mechanism. Arch Surg 117:675, 1982.
43. Jones TN, Moore EE, Van Way CW: Factors influencing nutritional assessment in abdominal trauma patients. JPEN 7:115, 1983.
44. Christou NV, Meakins JL: Delayed hypersensitivity in surgical patients—a mechanism for anergy. Surgery 33:322, 1978.

45. Moore EE, Dunn EL, Moore JB, et al: Penetrating abdominal trauma index. J Trauma 21:439, 1981.
46. Damask NC, Weissman C, Askanazi J, et al: A systematic method for validation of gas exchange measurements. Anesthesiology 57:213, 1982.
47. Ultman JS, Bursztein S: Analysis of error in the determination of respiratory gas exchange at varying FIO_2. J Appl Physiol 50:210, 1981.
48. Border JR, Chenier R, McMenamy RH, et al: Multiple systems organ failure: Muscle fuel deficit with visceral protein malnutrition. Surg Clin North Am 97:734, 1976.
49. Abel RM, Grimes JR, Alonso D, et al: Adverse hemodynamic and ultrastructural changes in dog hearts subjected to protein-calorie malnutrition. Am. Heart J 97:734, 1979.
50. Arora NS, Rochester DF: Respiratory muscle strength and maximal voluntary ventilation in undernourished patients. Am Rev Resp Dis 126:5.
51. Alverdy J, Chi HS, Sheldon GF: The effect of parenteral nutrition on gastrointestinal immunity. Ann Surg 202:681, 1985.
52. Kudsk KA, Carpenter G, Peterson S, et al: Effects of enteral and parenteral feeding in malnourished rats with *E. coli*-hemoglobin adjuvant peritonitis. J Surg Res 31:105, 1981.
53. Kudsk, KA, Stone JM, Carpenter G, et al: Enteral and parenteral feeding influences mortality after hemoglobin-*E. coli* peritonitis in normal rats. J Trauma 23:605, 1983.
54. Morchizuki H, Trocki O, Dominoni L, et al: Mechanism of prevention of postburn hypermetabolism and catabolism by early enteral feeding. Ann Surg 200:297, 1984.
55. Saito H, Trocki O, Alexander JW, et al: The effect of route of nutrient administration on the nutritional state, catabolic hormone secretion, and gut mucosal integrity after burn injury. JPEN 11:1, 1987.
56. Alexander W, MacMillian BG, Stinnett JD, et al: Beneficial effects of aggressive protein feeding in severely burned children. Ann Surg 192:505, 1980.
57. Page CP, Carlton PK, Adrassy RJ: Safe cost-effective postoperative nutrition— Defined formula diet via needle catheter jejunostomy. Am J Surg 138:939, 1979.
58. Moore EE, Dunn EL, Jones TJ: Immediate jejunostomy feeding: its use after major abdominal trauma. Arch Surg 116:681, 1981.
59. Moore EE, Jones TN: Benefits of immediate jejunostomy feeding after major abdominal trauma—a prospective randomized study. J Trauma 26:874, 1986.
60. Randall HT, Hooveer HC, Moore EE, et al: Nutritional support: enteral or parenteral. Contemp Surg 28:4, 1986.
61. Delany HM, Camevale NJ, Garvey JW: Jejunostomy by needle catheter technique. Surgery 73:786, 1973.
62. Hoover HC, Ryan JA, Anderson EJ, et al: Nutritional benefits of immediate postoperative jejunal feeding of an elemental diet. Am J Surg 139:153, 1980.

63. Jones TN, Moore FA, Moore EE, et al: Gastrointestinal symptoms attributed to jejunostomy feedings following major abdominal trauma. A critical analysis. Crit Care Med 17:1146–1150, 1989.
64. Ryan JA, Page CP: Intrajejunal feeding: development and current status. JPEN 8:198, 1984.
65. Wilmore DW, Smith RJ, O'Dwyer ST, et al: The gut—a central organ following surgical stress. Surgery 104:917, 1988.
66. Deitch EA, Maejima K, Berg R: Effect of oral antibiotics and bacterial overgrowth on the translocation of the GI tract microflora in burned rats. J Trauma 25:385, 1985.
67. Deitch EA, Winterton J, Berg R: The gut as a portal of entry for bacteremia. Ann Surg 205:681, 1987.
68. Wells CL, Rotstein OD, Pruett TL, et al: Intestinal bacteria translocate into experimental intraabdominal abscesses. Arch Surg 123:162, 1986.
69. Marshall JC, Lee C, Meakins JL, et al: Kupffer cell modulation of the systemic immune response. Arch Surg 122:191, 1987.
70. Revhag A, Michie HR, Manson JM, et al: Inhibition of cyclooxygenase attenuates the metabolic response to endotoxin in humans. Arch Surg 123:162, 1988.
71. Johnson LR, Copeland EM, Dudrick SJ, et al: Structural and hormonal alterations in the gastrointestinal tract of parenterally fed rats. Gastroenterology 68:1177, 1975.
72. Eastwood GL: Small bowel morphology and epithelial proliferation in intravenously alimented rabbits. Surgery 82:613, 1977.
73. Gimmon Z, Murphy RF, Chen MH, et al: The effect of parenteral and enteral nutrition on portal and systemic immunoreactivities of gastrin glucagon and vasoactive intestinal polypeptide (VIP). Arch Surg 196: 571, 1982.
74. Grant JP, Snyder BA: Use of L-glutamine in total parenteral nutrition. J Surg Res 44:506, 1988.
75. Moore FA, Moore EE, Jones TN, et al: TEN versus TPN following major torso injury—reduced septic morbidity. J Trauma 29:916, 1989.
76. Hurt AV, Ochsner JL, Schiller WR: Prolonged ileus after severe pelvic fracture. Am J Surg 146:755, 1983.
77. Cerra FB, Shronts EP, Konstantinides, NN: Enteral feeding in sepsis: a prospective randomized, double blind trial. Surgery 104:727, 1988.
78. Delany HM, Carnevale NJ, Garney JW: Jejunostomy by needle catheter technique. Surgery 73:786, 1973.
79. McArtle AH, Echave W, Brown RA, et al: Effect of elemental diet on pancreatic secretions. Am J Surg 128:690, 1974.
80. Cogbill TH, Wolfson RH, Moore EE, et al: Massive pneumatosis intestinalis and subcutaneous emphysema: complication of needle catheter jejunostomy. JPEN 7:171, 1983.
81. Hostetler C, Lipman TO, Geraghty M, et al: Bacterial safety of reconstructed continuous drip tube feedings. JPEN 6:232, 1982.

82. Schroeder P, Fisher F, Voltz M, et al: Microbial contamination of enteral feeding solutions in a community hospital. JPEN 7:364, 1983.
83. Steiger E, et al: Intravenous hyperalimentation: temporary and permanent vascular access and administration, in Deital (ed) Nutrition in Clinical Surgery. Baltimore: Williams and Wilkins, 1985.
84. Aubaniac R: L'injection intraveineuse sousclaviculair: avantages et téchnique. Presse Med 60:1456, 1952.
85. Jernigan WR, et al: Use of the internal jugular vein for placement of central venous catheters. Surg Gynecol Obstet 120:520, 1970.
86. Grimble GK, et al: Administration of fat emulsions with nutritional mixtures from the 3-liter delivery system in total parenteral nutrition. JPEN 9:456, 1985.
87. Hansen W: Fat tolerance and post heparin lipoprotein in liver disease. MMWR 117:841, 1975.
88. Abel RM: Nutritional support in the patient with acute renal failure. J Am Coll Nutr 2:33, 1983.
89. Sargent JA: Urea mass balance: nutrition and treatment of the acutely ill patient. Nutr Supp Serv 2:33, 1982.
90. Cerra FB, et al: Cirrhosis, encephalopathy, and improved results with metabolic support. Surgery 94:612, 1983.
91. Brennan MF, et al: Major contributor of the short term protein sparing effects of fat emulsions in normal man. Ann Surg 182:386, 1975.
92. Otamiri T: Oxygen radical, lipid peroxidation, and neutrophil infiltration after small intestinal ischemia and reperfusion. Surgery 105:593, 1988.
93. Meyer J, Yurt RW, Duhaney R, et al: Differential neutrophil activatid before and after endotoxin infusion in enterally versus parenterally fed volunteers. Surg Gynecol Obstet 167:501, 1988.
94. Wilmore D: The practice of clinical nutrition: how to prepare for the future. JPEN 13:337, 1989.
95. Hammerqvist F, Wernerman J, Ali R, et al: Addition of glutamine to total parenteral nutrition after elective abdominal surgery spares free glutamine in muscle, counteracts the fall in muscle protein synthesis, and improves nitrogen balance. Ann Surg 209:455, 1989.
96. Jacobs DO, Evans DA, Mealy K, et al: Combined effects of glutamine and epidermal growth factor in the rat intestine. Surgery 104:358, 1988.
97. Schwartz MZ, Storozuk RB: Influence of epidermal growth factor on intestinal function in the rat. Am J Surg 155:18, 1988.

Transition Feeding

CHAPTER 9

*Elaine Barbella Trujillo, M.S., R.D., CNSD
and Patricia M. Queen, M.Ms., R.D.*

INTRODUCTION

Transition feeding is the provision of nutrients when changing from one route of feeding to another or from one enteral product to another. Four modalities of transition feeding will be discussed in this chapter. They include the transition from parenteral nutrition (PN) to tube feeding (TF); PN to an oral diet; TF formula to TF formula; and TF to an oral diet.

Due to the high cost and numerous metabolic and mechanical complications associated with PN, it is highly desirable to make the transition from PN to enteral nutrition, as soon as is medically feasible. This is also desirable to preserve or improve gastrointestinal (GI) function. Disuse of the gut results in villous atrophy. Every 48 to 72 hr, the lining of the gastrointestinal tract is renewed. If there are inadequate nutrients to continue the turnover or if the gut is not used at all, there will be damage to the mucosal barrier. If the intestinal barrier is damaged, bacteria, endotoxin, viruses, and fungi inside the lumen of the gut can potentially move into the lymph nodes, bloodstream, and organs and lead to infection. This is commonly referred to as bacterial translocation (1). Parenteral nutrition has been associated with increased translocation, while translocation is decreased when nutrients are given enterally (2). Recent clinical investigation in nutrition support dictates that "if the gastrointestinal tract works it should be used" (3).

Patients on PN who are metabolically stable with a viable GI tract and no sings of GI intolerance are potential candidates for the transition to enteral intake. The clinician must keep in mind that the main concern in making the transition is the provision of adequate macro- and micronutrients. Before one changes a patient's diet from PN to enteral nutrition (EN), a reassessment of the patient's protein, calorie, and fluid requirements is necessary. During the progression, close monitoring of oral intake, GI tolerance, fluid balance, and nutritional assessment parameters are crucial in maintaining optimal metabolic and nutritional status. Calorie counts should be initiated once the patient is receiving a full liquid diet and is consuming at least 200 kCal/day. If nausea, vomiting, abdominal distention, diarrhea, and/or cramping are present, without any changes in medications or medical therapies, the diet progression or TF should be halted and the route of feeding reassessed. An assessment of the functional capacity of the gastrointestinal tract, the ability to take adequate oral intake, and the need for tube feedings are the first steps in the transitional process. A nomogram to assess the choices that must be made is included in Chapter 20.

PARENTERAL TO ENTERAL TUBE FEEDINGS

The assessment of tube feeding access is necessary before beginning enteral TF. In patients who are at risk of aspiration, the jejunal route is preferable. If, however, there is no concern regarding aspiration and the gag reflex is present, the gastric route may be used (4,5). The duration of tube feedings is also a criterion in selecting the appropriate feeding tube access. In patients who may require TF for at least 4 weeks, a permanently placed feeding tube is indicated (4,6).

The selection of an appropriate enteral formula is essential for successful transition to tube feeding. A prolonged period of no oral intake (NPO) (more than 1 week), recent GI surgery, or evidence of GI impairment are reasons to choose an elemental/predigested formula instead of a polymeric formula (4,7,8). Feedings should be initiated at 10–20 ml/hr and increased by 5–10 ml/hr every 8–12 hr until the desired rate is achieved (7). The PN rate should concomitantly decrease with the increase in rate of the TF formula. Formulas should be provided at full strength and not diluted. Rees et al. showed that an undiluted, hypertonic elemental diet, administered by continuous nasogastric infusion over 24 hr, was well tolerated by patients with impaired gastrointestinal function due to inflammatory bowel disease and the short bowel syndrome (9).

Patients without evidence of GI dysfunction can start with a polymeric, intact-protein enteral formula at 25 ml/he and this can be advanced by increments of 20 ml/hr every 12–24 hr to the desired rate while the PN rate is simultaneously decreased (4,7). Again, there is no need to dilute TF formulas since this may lead to hypocaloric regimens and negative nitrogen balance (9–11). It is preferable to begin TFs continuously via a pump. Cyclic or bolus feedings can be used once the patient is tolerating the goal volume of TF.

Close monitoring of GI symptoms is necessary throughout the transition period. Diarrhea is probably the most significant challenge in tube-fed patients, and fluid and electrolyte balances need to be watched carefully. The TF formulas are often blamed for causing diarrhea; however, this is generally not the case. There are numerous other potential causes of diarrhea, including use of antibiotics, sorbitol-containing medications (12), and other medications, such as magnesium antacids, cimetidine, potassium and phosphorus supplements, laxatives, and lactulose (11,13). In addition, hypoalbuminemia does not appear to be related to the incidence of diarrhea (11). If diarrhea does persist and other potential causes are ruled out, a low-fat formula may improve tolerance.

PARENTERAL NUTRITION TO ORAL INTAKE

PN to an Oral Diet

The decision to make the transition from PN to an oral diet depends primarily on the premise that the patient will progress to a full oral diet rapidly. The patient must have no evidence of malabsorption or maldigestion (14). In addition, the patient needs to be willing and motivated to eat by mouth.

The general practice is to initiate feedings with water or clear liquids, 30–60 ml at 20–30 min intervals and to increase the amount, depending on tolerance (4). Full liquids are usually begun on day 2 or once tolerance to clear liquids has been established, with the progression to soft or regular solids, usually by day 3.

Calorie counts should be completed and monitored daily. Once the patient is meeting 2/3 to 3/4 of protein and calorie requirements consistently, over a 3 day period, PN can be discontinued. The guideline of patients meeting 60% of caloric requirements has been established by Winkler et al. (15) to be acceptable for weaning from PN. This was evidenced by improved concentrations of all measured plasma proteins and maintenance of body weight in their patients.

Fluid balance should be managed closely throughout the transition period. As the patient increases oral consumption of liquids, the rate of PN should simultaneously be decreased.

Diet modification for fat, residue, and/or lactose may initially be indicated in patients with prolonged malnutrition and/or prolonged disease of the GI tract (14,16). Small, frequent feedings are also indicated in patients who complain of early satiety.

The clinician's role is crucial in making the transition from PN to oral intake successful. Encouraging the patient to eat nutrient-dense foods and beverages, including nutritional supplements, is often necessary. In addition, the fortification of foods and beverages with modular macronutrients, such as protein, carbohydrate, and fat sources, aids in optimizing nutrient intake.

PN to Oral Formula Diets

In some cases, the transition will occur from PN to oral formula diets. For example, oral intake from primarily nutritional supplements is indicated in patients with a viable GI tract but difficulty swallowing, such as those with head and neck carcinoma, patients with stroke, patients with ill-fitting dentures, and others. In these cases, the patient may benefit psychologically from this route of nutrition more than from the placement of a feeding tube.

In other cases, such as patients with inflammatory bowel disease or enteritis due to the acquired immunodeficiency syndrome (AIDS), in whom malabsorption and maldigestion may be likely, the transition to a low-fat, elemental formula may be indicated. Creative use of flavoring with juices, frozen concentrates, and various flavored beverages and/or the use of flavor packets (e.g., *Ross, Norwich Eaton*) is often necessary when using elemental formulas for oral consumption, since they are otherwise unpalatable (17). Recipe suggestions are also available from a variety of companies that produce enteral formulas.

Progression, as in oral food diets, is gradual, beginning with 30–60 ml and advancing according to the patients' tolerance. If the patient is unable to meet protein and caloric requirements within 5–7 days of initiating oral intake, reassessment of feeding tube placement may be necessary.

TRANSITION BETWEEN TF FORMULAS

Once the patient is off PN and stable on TF, it may be possible to make the transition to another enteral product. For example, this is often advantageous when using very expensive products or those requiring mixing. In addition, availability of some products is limited and switching to products that are available in local pharmacies may make the home TF process more convenient for the patient.

TF TO ORAL DIET

The initiation of oral intake should begin as soon as medically feasible unless there is evidence of mechanical difficulties with chewing and/or swallowing or the patient is disabled secondary to stroke, coma, or other conditions. Patients who have been NPO for a prolonged period of time, patients who have exhibited some form of GI intolerance on TFs, or patients who have undergone major intestinal surgery should make the transition to an oral diet slowly. Due to the high osmolality of clear liquid food items, it may be necessary to dilute to half strength (18). This is generally indicated in patients who have had extensive bowel resection and experience increased transit time. A summary of the osmolalities of food items on a clear liquid menu (and full menus) are listed in Table 9-1.

A patient eating only clear liquid diet usually progresses to receive a full liquid diet. However, full liquid diets are comprised primarily of dairy products and, therefore, tend to be high in fat and lactose. This may cause intolerance in patients with compromised gut function. This can be remedied by the addition of lactose-free supplements and/or advancement to a solid diet, which has greater variety. In addition, products such as *Lactaid* or *Ease* can be used by patients who are lactose intolerant. A low-fat diet is indicated in patients with a known fat intolerance. A suggested diet progression in patients with impaired gut function is as follows:

Day 1: 1/2-strength clear liquid diet

Day 2 (or as indicated): Full liquid diet with nutritional supplement of choice

Day 3 (or as indicated): Regular or therapeutic diet

Patients who do not exhibit signs of impaired gut function can begin on a full liquid diet with the addition of nutritional supplements, as needed. Once tolerance is established over 12–24 hr, the diet should be advanced to solid food.

Cyclic feeding is the provision of TF formula over a designated period. It is usually provided at night and is thought to increase the patient's appetite and allow for increased ambulation during the day. cyclic tube feedings should begin once the patient is eating solid food. A suggested cycling regimen is as follows:

Day 1: Cycle over 18 hr

Day 2: Decrease cycle to 12 hr

Day 3: Decrease cycle to 8 or 10 hr, or desired time period

As the cyclic time is decreased, the TF rate is increased to provide the desired volume. Because of the shortened TF infusion time, formulas are often concentrated to 1.5 or 2.0 kCal/ml.

TABLE 9-1. Beverage Osmolalities from Clear and Full Menus

Beverage	Mean Osmolalities (mOsm/kg)
Juices	
Prune	1076
Cranberry	836
Pineapple	772
Apple	705
Tomato	619
Grapefruit	618
Orange	601
V-8	578
Low-calorie cranberry	287
Broth	
Low-sodium, low-fat chicken	452
Regular chicken	389
Water ice	
Cherry	1064
Gelatin dessert	
Cherry	735
Low-calorie gelatin	57
Soft drinks	
Cola	714
Diet cola	43
Ginger ale	565
Diet ginger ale	53
Coffee/tea	
Tea	8
Tea with 1 teaspoon sugar	106
Tea with artificial sweetener	84
Coffee	33
Coffee with 1 teaspoon sugar	128
Coffee with artificial sweetener	114
Milk	
Whole milk	277
Skim milk	280
Lactaid with whole milk	413
Lactaid with skim milk	375
Carnation Instant Breakfast with whole milk	653
Carnation Instant Breakfast with skim milk	617
Carnation Instant Breakfast with whole Lactaid milk	723
Carnation Instant Breakfast with skim Lactaid milk	727

Source: Adapted from ref. 18.

Calorie counts and fluids should be monitored on a daily basis. Once the patient is consuming 2/3 or 3/4 of protein and energy needs, consistently over a 3 day period, the tube can be removed or, if permanent access has been installed, capped and flushed regularly to remain patent.

REFERENCES

1. Martindale RG, Andrassy RJ: Elemental nutrition overview. Reprinted from Nutritional Support Stategies for the Catabolic Patient. Proceedings from the American Dietetic Association Meeting, October 16–18, 1990, Denver, Colorado.
2. Bower RH: Nutrition and immune function. Nutr Clin Pract 5:189, 1990.
3. Rombeau JL, Caldwell MD (eds): Enteral and Tube Feeding. Philadelphia: WB Saunders, 1984.
4. Zibrida JM, Carlson S: Transitional feeding, in Shronts E (ed) Nutrition support Dietetics Core Curriculum. Rockville, MD: ASPEN Publishers, 1983.
5. Rombeau JD, Caldwell MD, Forlaw L, Guenter PA: Atlas of Nutritional Support Techniques. Boston: Little, Brown, 1989.
6. Monturo CA: Enteral access device selection. Nutr Clin Pract 5(5):207, 1990.
7. Paradis KM, Bell SJ, Benotti PN: Transitional feeding in small bowel resection, in Blackburn GL, Bell SJ, Mullen JL (eds) Nutritional Medicine: A Case Management Approach. Philadelphia, WB Saunders, 1989.
8. Bell SJ, Pasulka PS, Blackburn GL: Enteral formulas, in Skipper A (ed) Dietitian's Handbook of Enteral and Parenteral Nutrition. Rockville, MD: ASPEN Publishers, 1989.
9. Rees RGP, Keohane PP, Grimble GK, Frost PG, Attrill H, Silk DBA: Tolerance of elemental diet administered without starter regimen. Br Med J 290:1869, 1985.
10. Keohane PP, Attrill H, Love M, Frost P, Silk DBA: Relation between osmolality of diet and gastrointestinal side effects in enteral nutrition. Br Med J 288:678, 1984.
11. Gottschlich MM, Warden GD, Michel M, Havens P, Kopcha R, Jenkins M, Alexander JW: Diarrhea in tube-fed burn patients: incidence, etiology, nutritional impact, and prevention. JPEN 12(4):338, 1988.
12. Edes TE, Walk B, Austin JL: Diarrhea in tube-fed patients: feeding formula not necessarily the cause. Am J Med 88:91,1990.
13. Heimburger DC: Diarrhea with enteral feeding: will the real cause please stand up? Am J Med 88:89, 1990.
14. Wade, J: Parenteral and enteral transition techniques, in Krey SH, Murray RL (eds) Dynamics of Nutrition Support. Norwalk, CT: Appleton-Century-Crofts, 1986.
15. Winkler MF, Pomp A, Caldwell MD, Albina JE: Transitional feeding: the relationship between nutritional intake and plasma protein concentrations. J Am Diet Assoc 89(7):969, 1989.

16. Krey SH, Murray RL: Modular and transitional feedings, in Rombeau JL, Caldwell MD (eds) Enteral and Tube Feedings. Philadelphia, WB Saunders, 1990.
17. Rombeau JL, Caldwell MD (eds): Enteral and Tube Feeding. Philadelphia: WB Saunders, 1984.
18. Bell SJ, Anderson FL, Bistrian BR, Danner EH, Blackburn GL: Osmolality of beverages commonly provided on clear and full liquid menus. Nutr Clin Pract 2:241, 1987.

Selecting Enteral Products

CHAPTER 10

*Patrick S. Pasulka, M.D., F.A.C.P.
and Christine Crockett, R.D., CNSD*

An ever-expanding array of enteral feeding products is available for nutrition support. Selecting the appropriate formula to nourish optimally the acutely or chronically ill patient challenges even experienced nutritionists. Formulas are often selected based on the hospital's contract, prescriber's preference and habit, and marketing efforts by suppliers. Many currently available formulas have been designed based on sound theoretical principles. However, few scientific comparisons of formulas have been performed under clinical conditions. This chapter focuses on clinical decision making, based on theory and science, for the appropriate selection of categories of enteral products. Although manufacturers may choose to emphasize the advantages of a particular product within a given category, the following discussion will largely avoid such comparisons.

CHOOSING ENTERAL PRODUCTS

Initial Assessment

In addition to assessing the patient's nutritional status and the integrity of the gastrointestinal tract, a clinical assessment of the patient's pertinent medical problems will aid in the selection of the feeding product. This assessment includes evaluating for electrolyte imbalances, diabetes, congestive heart failure, pancreatic insufficiency, renal insufficiency, liver disease and lung disease, and the presence and severity of catabolic stressors. Once the initial assessment is complete, the appropriate formula can usually be selected by asking a series of eight questions.

Figure 10-1 shows the components involved in this decision.

Does the Patient Have Maldigestion?

Predigested formulas, including elemental, chemically defined, and peptide-based formulas, require little or not digestion for their absorption. The original Vivonex (now Tolerex, Norwich Eaton) is the prototype (1) of these formulas and consists of free amino acids, glucose and oligosaccharides, and a small amount of safflower oil. Several partially hydrolyzed formulas consisting of short-chain polypeptides and hydrolyzed starches were subsequently designed. These are not as elemental, but appear to be absorbed with equal or greater facility (2,3). Most recently, formulas providing a high proportion of protein as di- and tripeptides have been developed (Reabilan, O'Brien Pharmaceuticals) with the theoretical advantage of employing a separate intestinal transport system, thus facilitating protein absorption (4,5).

Predigested formulas are ideal for patients with maldigestion, such as those with pancreatic insufficiency or with biliary or pancreatic diversion (6). They may also be useful in situations of malabsorption, as occurs in patients with sprue or short-bowel syndrome (7). These formulas have been tested for their use in acute exacerbations of Crohn's disease, with some promise that they may be effective first-line therapy (8-12). Other studies suggest that the accrued benefit may be due to the improvement in overall nutritional status rather than to the elemental nature of these formulas (13-15).

Elemental and peptide-based formulas are often marketed for their efficiency of absorption in the setting of early post operative feeding. The nitrogen may be absorbed more efficiently than that of whole protein, but net nitrogen balance may not differ. Predigested formulas are also marketed for the treatment of diarrhea associated with enteral feeding. Such diarrhea is multifactorial and is often not amenable to elemental diets. Nevertheless it is useful to try one of these formulas when the diarrhea is resistant to other measures (16,17) This is discussed in more detail at the end of this chapter.

Table 10-1 lists currently available predigested formulas.

Does the Patient Have Liver Disease?

Early in the development of parenteral nutrition, Fisher and his colleagues at the Massachusetts General Hospital noticed consistently abnormal serum amino

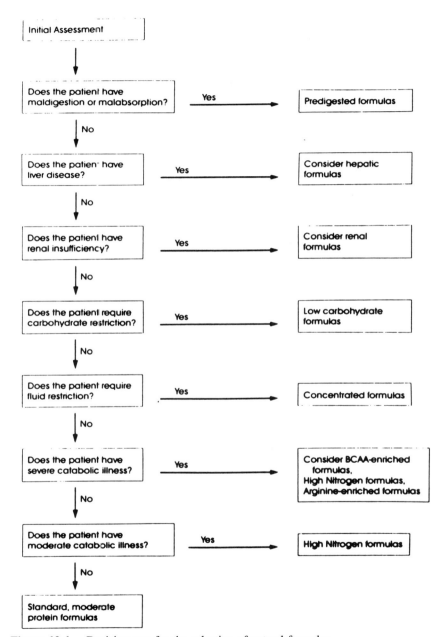

Figure 10-1. Decision tree for the selection of enteral formulas.

TABLE 10-1. Predigested Formulas

	kCal/ml	G Protein/ 1000 kCal	Protein Source	G Fat/ 1000 kCal	kCal to meet RDA	Na$^+$–K$^+$/ 1000 kCal	mOsm
Acupep HPF (Sherwood Med)	1.0	40	Hydrolyzed lactalbumin	10	1600	30-29	490
Criticare HN (Mead Johnson)	1.06	36	Hydrolyzed casein/free AAs	3.2	2000	26-32	650
Peptamin (Clintec)	1.0	40	Hydrolyzed whey	39	1500	22-32	270
Pepti-2000 (Sherwood Med)	1.0	40	Hydrolyzed lactalbumin	10	1600	30-30	490
Reabilin (O'Brien)	1.0	31.5	Whey and casein peptides	43	2250	31-32	350
Reabilin HN (O'Brien)	1.33	43.6	Whey and casein peptides	43	2500	33-32	490
Tolerex (Norwich Eaton)	1.0	20.6	Free AAs	1.4	1800	20-30	550
Travasorb (Clintec)	1.0	30	Hydrolyzed lactalbumin	13.5	2000	40-30	560
Travasorb HN (Clintec)	1.0	45	Hydrolyzed lactalbumin	13.5	2000	40-30	560
Vital HN (Ross)	1.0	41.7	Hydrolyzed whey soy, meat, and free AAs	10.8	1500	25-36	460
Vivonex TEN (Norwich Eaton)	1.0	38.2	Free AAs	2.8	2000	20-20	630

acid profiles among patients with liver disease (18, 19). Patients with chronic hepatic disease have elevated levels of methionine, glutamate, and the aromatic amino acids (AAA) tryptophan, phenylalanine, and tyrosine, and they have depressed levels of the branched-chain amino acids (BCAA) leucine, isoleucine, and valine. These investigators found an inverse relationship between the ratio of BCAA/AAA and the level of hepatic encephalopathy. Formulas enriched in BCAA were designed subsequently to normalize the ratio of BCAA/AAA in the plasma.

There have been several trials of branched-chain-enriched parenteral nutrition formulas, and their results have recently been analyzed using the technique of meta-analysis (20). Most experts agree that there are measurable benefits attributable to the provision of intravenous BCAA-enriched amino acids in the setting of hepatic encephalopathy.

Data pertaining to enteral formulas are less clear. McGhee (21) compared a 50 g casein protein diet with a 20 g casein/30 g Hepatic-Acid protein diet in four patients with known protein-intolerant hepatic insufficiency, in a nonblinded, crossover study. The ratio of BCAA/AAA increased significantly in patients on the Hepatic-Aid diet, but plasma ammonia levels did not change. Parameters of hepatic encephalopathy were not measurably altered on either dietary regimen.

Horst and colleagues (22) studied 37 patients with known cirrhosis and dietary protein intolerance, in a randomized, multicenter, double-blinded study. All patients began on a 20 g mixed protein diet. After the first week, 20 g of additional protein was added each week, to a total of 80 g/day. The control group received the additional protein as a mixed protein diet, the study group received the final 60 g of protein as a BCAA-enriched amino acid solution (A662, McGaw). Plasma BCAA levels increased in the study group; plasma ammonia did not change, nor did findings on the electroencephalogram. There were significant differences in mental status grade and in the portal–systemic encephalopathy index (PSEI). Seven of 20 patients in the control group developed stage II or greater coma, compared to only 1 of 17 in the BCAA group.

Christie et al. (23) examined a similar group of eight patients with known cirrhosis and protein intolerance in a randomized, double-blind, crossover study. Beginning with a 40 g protein, meat-free diet, the patients were given increments of either Ensure (casein-based) or Travasorb-Hepatic (BCAA-enriched) protein. Ultimately the patients received about 30 g of nonmeat dietary protein and approximately 45 g of the supplemental protein. The BCAA/AAA ratio increased while patients were on the BCAA-enriched supplement, but there was no detectable difference in the Reitan number connection test on either dietary regimen. The PSEI improved slightly on the casein-based supplement, but not on the BCAA-enriched supplement.

Egberts et al. (24) treated patients with latent portal–systemic encephalopathy with casein or branched-chain amino acid supplements in pill form, in a double-blind crossover study. Subtle benefits in psychometric testing were attributable to BCAAs, even though patients were not clinically encephalopathic.

Thus, BCAA-enriched enteral formulas appear to be superior to mixed dietary protein, but are not dramatically superior to standard casein-based enteral formulas, as measured by parameters of hepatic encephalopathy. This is not entirely unexpected. Prior to the development of disease-specific formulas, milk protein was the preferred protein source for patients with hepatic encephalopathy. In 1958, Bessman and colleagues (25) demonstrated that plasma ammonia levels were dramatically higher after volunteers ingested whole blood than after they ingested a casein-based protein formula. In 1966, Fenton et al. (26) showed stepped increases in plasma ammonia levels when patients progressed from dairy protein to vegetable protein to meat protein. Thus, of all natural protein sources, casein appears to be the least likely to precipitate or aggravate encephalopathy. Branched-chain-enriched formulas may be slightly superior to casein-based formulas in resolving encephalopathy.

A major advantage of the hepatic formulas is their low electrolyte content. Often patients with severe liver disease have ascites and are on potassium-sparing diuretics, so a low sodium and potassium content can be advantageous. On the other hand, because one of these formulas (Hepatic-Aid, McGaw) has no micronutrients, these have to be added separately. Appropriate use of these formulas requires significant nutritional expertise.

Table 10-2 lists formulas designed for patients with hepatic disease.

Does the Patient Have Renal Insufficiency?

In an attempt to reduce the production of nitrogenous wastes in the setting of acute or chronic renal failure, investigators in the 1970s designed protein formulas consisting of only essential amino acids (EAA) (27, 28). The body could theoretically recycle waste nitrogen to synthesize nonessential amino acids. However, there appears to be little recycling of urea nitrogen, (29). In trials of parenteral EAAs in patients with acute renal failure (30) or chronic renal insufficiency (31), there appears to be no advantage gained by these formulas. Essential amino acid formulas are adequate for net protein anabolism, but that is not synonymous with being an optimal protein source. In growing animals, a balanced amino acid formula results in better protein synthesis than an EAA formula (32). It is likely this also is true in the setting of catabolic illness.

No studies comparing EAA *enteral* formulas to standard enteral formulas have been published.

The value of these formulas lies in their low electrolyte content and high concentration of calories. It is common for patients with renal failure to have multiple electrolyte abnormalities, including hyperkalemia, hyponatremia or hypernatremia, hypercalcemia, hyperphosphatemia, and hypermagnesemia. One of

TABLE 10-2. Hepatic Formulas

	kCal/ml	G Prot/ 1000 kCal	kCal to meet RDA	Na^+-K^+/ 1000 kCal	mOsm	%BCAA
Hepatic Aid (McGaw)	1.2	37.5	0	<15-0	560	40
Travasorb Hepatic (Clintec)	1.1	26.7	2040	9.2-20.5	600	50

these formulas (Amin-Aid, McGaw) affords the opportunity to customize levels of electrolytes, minerals, and vitamins.

Urinary excretion is a major route of micronutrient elimination, so it is difficult to predict micronutrient requirements of patients with acute or chronic renal failure. In the short term, there is little harm in daily doses of vitamins and minerals. Doses three times weekly may be sufficient for long-term enterally fed patients. Monitoring vitamin and mineral levels or their functional end points may be necessary. In this era of recombinant erythropoietin, iron and vitamin deficiencies may become more obvious as inadequate erythropoiesis.

By current standards, the renal formulas are low in protein content. If it is desirable to use these formulas for their electrolyte advantages, the protein concentration can be supplemented with a casein or egg white protein powder. This will result in an EAA-enriched protein with high biological value.

Table 10-3 lists the enteral formulas designed for patients with renal failure.

Does the Patient Require Carbohydrate Restriction?

Pulmonary formulas. Based on work by Askanazi and Kinney (33, 34), it is evident that excessive feeding of carbohydrate can result in increased production of carbon dioxide, potentially precipitating respiratory failure in susceptible patients.

The respiratory quotient (RQ) is the ratio of carbon dioxide produced (VCO_2) to oxygen consumed (VO_2) during the oxidation of a substrate. Different substrates oxidize at different RQs: lipid oxidation has an RQ of 0.70; protein oxidation has an RQ of 0.80; carbohydrate oxidation has an RQ of 1.00. Thus, the oxidation of carbohydrate results in more CO_2 production than the oxidation of lipid. Lipogenesis from carbohydrate has an RQ in excess of 2.5. Thus there is an energy and carbon dioxide cost of excessive carbohydrate feeding. Pulmocare (Ross Labs) was developed to provide a greater percentage of nonprotein calories as lipid instead of carbohydrate for enteral feeding in the setting of ventilatory insufficiency.

Serog (35) performed a study comparing four parenteral formulas resembling commercially available enteral products, fed to burn patients. The patients were fed according to their measured energy requirements. There was a significant increase in the measured RQ on the high-carbohydrate formula compared to the high-lipid formula. There was little difference in RQs between the standard 2:1 carbohydrate/lipid formula and the 1:2 carbohydrate/lipid formula.

Heymsfield et al. (36) demonstrated increased carbon dioxide production, increased heat production, and increased minute ventilation from high-carbohydrate (83% of total calories) feedings compared to high-fat (50% of total calories) feedings.

TABLE 10-3. Renal Formulas

	kCal/ml	G Prot/ 1000 kCal	kCal to meet RDA	Na$^+$–K$^+$/ 1000 kCal	mOsm	%EAA
AminAid (McGaw)	2.0	10	0	<8-0	700	100
Replena (Ross)	2.0	14.9	1920	392-558	615	NA
Travasorb Renal (Clintec)	1.4	17	0	0-0	590	60

Al-Saady et al. (37) studied two small groups of ventilated patients fed with either Pulmocare or Ensure Plus. They were able to demonstrate a fall in PCO_2 in the Pulmocare-fed group, and a significantly shorter time to weaning. The study consisted of only 20 patients, so the results should be considered preliminary.

Kane et al. (38) fed 10 young adults with cystic fibrosis, with a mean baseline PCO_2 of 53, night-time enteral infusions of Pulmocare, Ensure Plus, or Vivonex TEN. The RQ increased progressively with each of the formulas (0.88, 1.00, and 1.08, respectively) as did the VCO_2 (174, 197, and 206 ml/min/m^2, respectively) and the minute ventilation (6.54, 6.72, and 7.37 L/min/m^2 respectively). However, PCO_2 did not increase appreciably. Thus, measurable differences in carbon dioxide production were evident, but even these patients with carbon dioxide retention were able to compensate adequately.

There has been concern in the scientific literature about the potential adverse effects of excessive intravenous lipid, but these enteral studies have not demonstrated any adverse effects of the high-lipid enteral formulas. Mochizuki et al. (39) demonstrated less carcass weight, less muscle mass, and lower transferrin levels in burned guinea pigs fed high-fat diets (30–50% lipid) than in those fed low-fat enteral diets (5–15% lipid), but otherwise there are not documented adverse effects of high-lipid enteral formulas.

Diabetes formulas. During the clinical use of Pulmocare, it became evident that a low-carbohydrate formula facilitated glucose control in diabetic or insulin-resistant patients. This led to the development of a low-carbohydrate formula for use in diabetic patients (Glucerna, Ross Labs). This formula provides 50% of the total calories as lipid (70% monounsaturated) and 33% as carbohydrate (21% of carbohydrate as fructose). Peters et al. (40) demonstrated significantly less glucose elevation when this formula (EN-8715) was compared to Ensure HN. This low-carbohydrate formula is likely to be most useful in the setting of severe insulin resistance.

Table 10-4 lists the currently available low-carbohydrate formulas.

Is the Patient Fluid Restricted?

Many patients who require enteral feeding are not able to tolerate large amounts of fluid. Standard formulas provide 1.0–1.2 kCal/ml. Most enteral products are 75–85% free water. Feeding 2000 calories of standard formulas can provide 1500–1700 ml water per day. Patients with congestive heart failure, ascites, oliguric renal insufficiency, or pulmonary edema require fluid-restricted formulas. The more concentrated enteral formulas are similar in composition to standard formulas but provide either 1.5 or 2.0 kCal/ml. The water content of these formulas is 65–75% by volume. Table 10-5 lists concentrated formulas.

TABLE 10-4. Carbohydrate-Restricted Formulas

	kCal/ml	G Prot/ 1000 kCal	G Fat/1000 kCal	G CHO/ 1000 kCal	kCal to meet RDA	Na^+-K^+/ 1000 kCal	mOsm
Glucerna (Ross)	1.0	41.8	55.7	93.7	1422	40-40	375
Pulmocare (Ross)	1.5	41.7	61.4 (55%) Corn oil	70.4	1420	38-29.5	490

TABLE 10-5. Concentrated Formulas

	kCal/ml	G Protein/ 1000 kCal	G Fat/ 1000 kCal	kCal to meet RDA	Na$^+$–K$^+$/ 1000 kCal	mOsm
Comply (Sherwood)	1.5	40	40	1500	32-32	410
Ensure Plus (Ross)	1.5	36.6	35.5	2130	31-33	690
Ensure Plus HN (Ross)	1.5	41.7	33.2	1420	34-33	650
Nutren 1.5 (Clintec)	1.5	40	45	1500	22-32	410
PulmoCare (Ross)	1.5	41.7	61.4	1420	38-30	490
Resource Plus (Sandoz)	1.5	36	35	2400	25-29	600
Sustacol HC (Mead Johnson)	1.5	40	39	1800	25-25	650
TraumaCal (Mead Johnson)	1.5	55	45.3	3000	34-24	490
IsoCal HCN (Mead Johnson)	2.0	37.4	51	2000	17-22	690
Magnacal (Sherwood)	2.0	35	40	2000	22-16	590
Nutren 2.0 (Clintec)	2.0	40	53	1500	22-32	710
TwoCal HN (Ross)	2.0	41.7	45.3	1600	29-31	690

Does the Patient Have Severe Catabolic Illness: Trauma, Burn, or Sepsis?

Branched-chain stress formulas. In severely hypercatabolic conditions, branched-chain amino acids are consumed as energy sources locally in the skeletal muscle, and are relatively depleted in the circulating amino acid pool. Investigators reasoned that formulas enriched with branched-chain amino acids would "normalize" the amino acid profile and might improve protein synthesis. Animal and human studies have demonstrated small increments in net protein synthesis (41–45) when BCAA-enriched parenteral formulas are used. It is not yet clear that a *clinical* benefit is attributable to this slightly improved nitrogen balance (46). The branched-chain content of these formulas is approximately 45% of total amino acids, as compared to approximately 21% for standard formulas. The Federation of American Societies for Experimental Biology's (47) consensus report on enteral products suggests that these formulas may benefit patients with prolonged hypercatabolic illnesses. The American Society for Parenteral and Enteral Nutrition (48) issued a consensus statement in 1986 to the effect that the use of branched-chain enriched formulas in the setting of hypercatabolic illness should still be considered investigational.

Cerra's study (44) provides the only available human data pertaining to enteral intake of branched-chain enriched formulas. Mochizuki et al. (46) found no benefit from branched-chain enriched feedings in their burned guinea pig model.

Immune-enhancing formulas. Two enteral products have recently been released that are intriguing because of their theoretical advantages. Sandoz Nutrition developed a product (Impact) supplemented with arginine (25% of amino acids) and nucleic acids, which have been demonstrated to stimulate in vivo and in vitro measures of immune function (49–52). It also contains a spectrum of fatty acids, including omega-3 fatty acids, mono- and poly-unsaturated fatty acids, and medium-chain fatty acids. Preliminary data suggest that this formula may have a clinical benefit in reducing patient morbidity and hospital stay (53). McGaw has since marketed a related formula (ImmunAid) that is also glutamine supplemented. Impact is currently the subject of a large prospective, multicenter trial.

Table 10-6 lists enteral products designed for hypercatabolic patients.

Does the Patient Require Extra Protein?

Standard enteral formulas are the time-honored first choice for initiating feedings. Over the past decade it has been recognized that calorie needs during catabolic illness are less than previously estimated. Reducing the total calories provided with standard formulas, however, reduces the protein below an acceptable level. For example, a moderately ill 70 kg patient may require 30 kCal/kg

TABLE 10-6. Trauma/Burn/Sepsis Formulas

	kCal/ml	G Prot/ 1000 kCal	kCal to meet RDA	Na$^+$–K$^+$/ 1000 kCal	mOsm	%BCAA
ImmunAid (McGaw)	1.0	80	2000	17-35	580	25
Impact (Sandoz)	1.0	56	1500	47-33	375	17
Stresstein (Sandoz)	1.2	58	2400	23-23	910	44
Traum Aid HBC (McGaw)	1.0	56	3000	23-30	675	50

or 2100 kCal/day. However, 2100 kCal of a standard formula would provide approximately 80 g protein/day or 1.1 g/kg. A daily protein goal is generally considered to be 1.5 g/kg for patients with moderate or severe catabolic illness. In the setting of catabolic illness, formulas with higher protein concentrations are recommended (54,55).

The division between standard protein formulas and high-protein formulas is somewhat arbitrary. Table 10-7 lists all the commercially available formulas with nonprotein calorie/nitrogen ratios less than 120:1, or those with more than 43 g protein/1000 kCal.

Does the Patient Require Long-Term, Maintenance Feeding?

For patients who are not acutely ill, and who are unlikely to benefit from the special formulas above, standard formulas can be used. These are ideal for long-term nutritional support, as provided in extended care facilities or enterally fed patients at home. Several manufacturers have developed fiber-containing formulas to reduce the diarrhea sometimes associated with enteral feeding, and to reduce the constipation sometimes associated with low-residue diets. There are several theoretical benefits to the addition of fiber to enteral formulas, including improvement of bowel function, availability of short-chain fatty acids to the colonic mucosa, and improved glucose tolerance curves. The major potential disadvantage of fiber is interference with mineral absorption (56–58). Several studies have looked at the relative value of fiber (57–65). These studies suggest a minor advantage to fiber-containing formulas in reducing constipation and increasing fecal water content. There does not appear to be an advantage in reducing diarrhea associated with tube feeding which is often related to antibiotics, diarrhea-inducing medications, or intrinsic intestinal pathologic conditions. There are few objective data to support the use of fiber-containing over non-fiber-containing formulas. For complete recent reviews of this subject see work by Palacio and Rombeau (66) Scheppach et al. (67), and Silk (68).

Table 10-8 lists the standard, moderate-protein formulas.

Summary

The science of enteral nutrition has lagged behind the marketplace. We hope that specific data pertaining to the appropriate use of disease-specific formulas will be forthcoming. In the meantime, this decision tree is intended to identify formally the intellectual process that should occur in the choice of a particular product.

TABLE 10-7. High-Nitrogen Formulas

	kCal/ml	G Prot/ 1000 kCal	G Fat/ 1000 kCal	kCal to meet RDA	Na$^+$-K$^+$/ 1000 kCal	mOsm	G TDF[a]
Entrition HN (Biosearch)	1.0	44	41	1300	40-41	300	—
Fibersource HN (Sandoz)	1.2	44	34.6	1800	26-36	390	6.8
ImmunAid (McGaw)	1.0	80	22	2000	17-35	580	—
Impact (Sandoz)	1.0	56	28	1500	47-33	375	—
IsoSource HN (Sandoz)	1.2	44	33	1800	26-36	330	—
Isotein HN (Sandoz)	1.2	57	28.6	2100	33-22	300	—
Meritene (Sandoz)	0.96	60	33.3	1124	40-43	510	—
Newpak HN (O'Brien KMI)	1.24	48.4	32.3	1550	30-30	310	—
Newtrition HN (O'Brien KMI)	1.24	48	28.6	1250	20-20	310	—
Newtrition Isofiber (O'Brien KMI)	1.18	43.2	32.1	1475	31-28	310	14.3
Replete (Clintec)	1.0	62	33	1500	22-40	350	—
Stresstein (Sandoz)	1.2	58	23	2400	23-23	910	—
Traumacal (Mead Johnson)	1.5	55	45.3	3000	24-24	490	—
TraumAid HBC (Kendall McGaw)	1.0	56	126	3000	23-30	675	—

[a]Total digestable fiber/1000 kCal.

THE PATIENT WITH DIARRHEA

Dysfunction of the gastrointestinal tract, especially distention and diarrhea, often prompts the decision to change formulas. From the literature, there does not appear to be a single "correct" response to this problem (69). Again, the problem should be approached systematically, as described in Figure 10-2. This discussion assumes that the patient does not have a known pre-existing intestinal disorder, such as gluten enteropathy, short-bowel syndrome, inflammatory bowel disease, or radiation enteritis.

Definition of Diarrhea

Gastrointestinal intolerance of enteral feedings, particularly diarrhea, is frequently observed in the clinical setting. Clinical surveys suggest that 1:3 or 1:4 patients will be troubled with loose stools while on enteral feeding (70, 71). Stooling is often more of a nursing hygiene problem than a true medical complication. Some attempt should be made to quantitate diarrhea. Clinically significant diarrhea can be arbitrarily defined as more than 300 ml liquid stool/day more than four loose bowel movements per day, or liquid stools that increase the risk of bacterial contamination (of indwelling urinary catheters, intravenous lines, decubitus ulcers, or surgical wounds).

Is There Blood in the Stool?

The first question is whether the stool contains occult blood. The presence of heme in the stool should prompt appropriate gastrointestinal work-up, including stool cultures, assays for *Clostridium difficile* toxin, and contrast studies or endoscopy, as indicated by the clinical situation.

Are Medications a Possible Cause?

Medications are the most common causes of diarrhea in enterally fed patients. Several studies have indicated that diarrhea with enteral feedings is most frequently associated with antibiotics (69, 70). It is appropriate to assay stool samples for *Clostridium difficile* toxin in any patient with diarrhea who has recently been taking antibiotics. However, antibiotics can be associated with diarrhea even in the absence of *C. difficile*. Many medications given as suspensions are provided in sorbitol suspensions. This nondigestible sugar-alcohol can cause osmotic diarrhea. A careful review of medications and a call to the pharmacy can often resolve this problem. Other medications that may cause diarrhea include magnesium-containing antacids, hypermotility agents (metoclopramide and macrolide antibiotics), quinidine, and aminophylline. Patients are also often

TABLE 10-8. Moderate-Nitrogen Standard Formulas

	kCal/ml	G Prot/ 1000 kCal	G Fat/ 1000 kCal	kCal to meet RDA	Na$^+$–K$^+$/ 1000 kCal	mOsm	G TDF
Attain (Sherwood)	1.0	40	35	1250	35-41	300	—
Complete Modified (Sandoz)	1.07	40	35	1605	41-33	300	4.3
Comply (Sherwood)	1.5	40	40	1500	32-32	500	—
Enrich (Ross)	1.1	36.2	33.9	1530	34-39	480	14.3
Ensure (Ross)	1.06	35.2	35.2	2000	35-38	470	—
Ensure HN (Ross)	1.06	42	33.6	1400	38-32	470	—
Ensure Plus HN (Ross)	1.5	41.7	33.2	1420	34-31	650	—
Entrition RDA (Biosearch)	1.0	36	35	1500	35-34	300	—
Fibersource (Sandoz)	1.2	35	34	1800	20-30	390	10
Glucerna (Ross)	1.0	41.8	55.7	1422	40-40	375	14.3
Isocal HN (Mead Johnson)	1.06	41.6	43	1250	33-26	300	—
Isocal (Mead Johnson)	1.06	32.5	42	2000	22-32	300	—
Isosource (Sandoz)	1.2	35	34	1800	26-36	360	—
Jevity (Ross)	1.06	42	34.8	1400	38-38	310	14.3
Newpak Isotonic (O'Brien KMI)	1.06	37.7	34	1325	28-28	300	—
Newtrition Isotonic (O'Brien KMI)	1.08	33.3	37	1325	24-24	300	—
Nutren (Clintec)	1.0	40	38	1500	22-32	300	—
Nutren 1.5 (Clintec)	1.5	40	45	1500	22-32	410	—

Nutren 2.0 (Clintec)	2.0	40	53	1500	22-32	710	—
Osmolite (Ross)	1.06	35.2	36.4	2000	26-24	300	—
Osmolite HN (Ross)	1.06	42	34.8	1400	38-38	300	—
Profiber (Sherwood)	1.0	40.1	40	1500	32-32	300	12.0
Pulmocare (Ross)	1.5	41.7	61.4	1420	38-30	490	—
Resource (Sandoz)	1.06	35	35	2010	35-38	450	—
Sustacal (Mead Johnson)	1.06	43	33.2	1500	30-34	450	5.9
VitaNeed (Sherwood)	1.0	40	40	1500	30-32	300	8.0
UltraCal (Mead Johnson)	1.06	41.5	42.3	1605	38-39	300	14.1

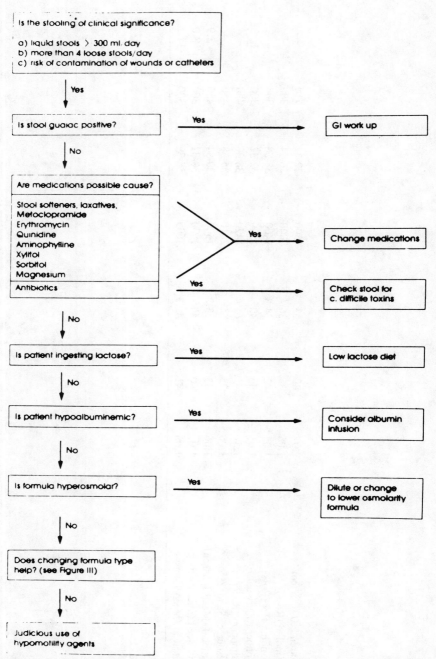

Figure 10-2. Approach to the patients with tube feeding associated diarrhea.

prescribed stool softeners or laxatives early in their course of therapy, and their use is inadvertently continued despite diarrhea.

Is the Patient Ingesting Lactose?

During the acute phases of illness, many patients lose their ability to digest lactose. Most commercially available enteral products do not contain lactose. When patients begin oral diets, especially full-liquid diets, lactose is reintroduced, resulting in osmotic diarrhea. A low-lactose diet may be all that is required for a patient in this situatiom.

Is the Patient Hypoalbuminemic?

It has recently been suggested that in the presence of low plasma albumin levels, improving serum osmolarity with the use of exogenous albumin may reduce the incidence of diarrhea (72). Not all authorities agree that this use of albumin is effective, and low plasma albumin levels are not universally associated with intolerance to enteral feeding (73).

Is the Enteral Formula Hyperosmolar?

Another potential cause of diarrhea is hyperosmolality of enteral products, although most products are well within the range of tolerable osmolarities. Several studies call into question the assumption that hyperosmolarity of enteral products induces diarrhea (74, 75). If the patient is receiving a formula with an osmolarity greater than 500 mOsm, changing to a formula with a lower osmolarity may be useful.

Does Changing the Type of Formula Help?

Once consideration is given to these possible causes of intolerance to enteral feeding, it is appropriate to change the enteral formula. No single formula is associated with a lower incidence of diarrhea. If one type of formula is not tolerated, it is advisable to switch to another category. The author uses the approach described in Figure 10-3. If a standard formula is poorly tolerated, it is advisable to change to a fiber-containing formula, and vice versa. If this is not effective in controlling the diarrhea, an elemental or peptide-based formula may be tried.

Will Hypomotility Agents Help?

If no treatable source of diarrhea can be discovered, hypomotility agents may be judiciously used. There is the obvious risk of masking a serious gastrointestinal problem, including infection, incomplete obstruction, or ischemia. Loperamide

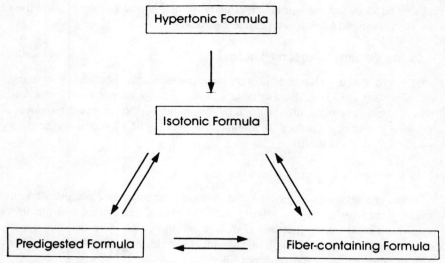

Figure 10-3. Suggested sequence of formula change, for tube feeding associated diarrhea.

hydrochloride, diphenoxylate hydrochloride/atropine sulfate, paregoric, codeine, and tincture of opiate are the most commonly used hypomotility agents.

SUMMARY

Understanding the theory and science of different categories of enteral feeding products affords the physician and the nutritionist the opportunity to make educated choices. Nutrition support has advanced beyond the simple provision of protein and calories. We have entered the era of nutritional pharmacology, and have the ability to have an incremental impact on the outcome of seriously ill patients by manipulating the balance of nutrients.

REFERENCES

1. Stephens RV, Randall HT: Use of a concentrated, balanced, liquid elemental diet for nutritional management of catabolic states. Ann Surg 170:642–667, 1969.
2. Feller AG, Caindec N, Rudman IW, Rudman D: Effects of three liquid diets on nutrition sensitive plasma proteins of tube-fed elderly men. J Am Geriatr Soc 38:663–668, 1990.

3. Trocki O, Mochizuki J, Dominioni L, Alexander JW: Intact protein versus free amino acids in the nutritional support of thermally injured animals. JPEN 10:139–145, 1986.
4. Ziegler F, Ollivier JM, Cynober L, et al: Efficiency of enteral nitrogen support in the surgical patients: small peptides v. non-degraded proteins. Gut 31:1277–1283, 1990.
5. Meredith JW, Ditesheim JA, Zaloga GP: Visceral protein levels in trauma patients are greater with peptide diet than with intact protein diet. J Trauma 30:825–829, 1990.
6. Steinhardt HJ, Wolf A, Jokober B, et al: Nitrogen absorption in pancreatectomized patients: protein versus protein hydrolysate as substrate. J Lab Clin Med 113:162–167, 1989.
7. Voitk AJ, Echabe B, Brown RA, Gurd FN: Use of elemental diet during the adaptive stage of short gut syndrome. Gastroenterology 65:419–426, 1973.
8. Belli DC, Seidman E, Bouthillier L, et al: Chronic intermittent elemental diet improves growth failure in children with Crohn's disease. Gastroenterology 94:603–610, 1988.
9. Giaffer MH, North G, Holdsworth CD: Controlled trial of polymeric versus elemental diet in treatment of active Crohn's disease. Lancet 335:816–819, 1990.
10. Morin CL, Roulet M, Roy CC, et al: Continuous elemental enteral alimentation in the treatment of children and adolescents with Crohn's disease. JPEN 6:194–199, 1982.
11. O'Morain C, Segal AW, Levi AJ: Elemental diets in treatment of acute Crohn's disease. Br Med J 281:1173–1175, 1980.
12. Sanderson IR, Udeen S, Davies PSW, et al: Remission induced by an elemental diet in small bowel Crohn's disease. Arch Dis Child 61:123–127, 1987.
13. Harries AD, Danis V, Heatley RV, et al: Controlled trial of supplemented oral nutrition in Crohn's disease. Lancet 887–890, 1983.
14. Greenberg GR, Fleming CR, Jeejeebhoy KN, et al: Controlled trial of bowel rest and nutritional support in the management of Crohn's disease. Gut 29:1309–1315, 1988.
15. Afdhal NH, Kelly J, McCormick PA, O'Donoghue DP: Remission induction in refractory Crohns disease using a high calorie whole diet. JPEN 13:362–365, 1989.
16. Brinson RR, Kolts BE: Diarrhea associated with severe hypoalbuminemia: a comparison of a peptide-based chemically defined diet and standard enteral alimentation. Crit Care Med 16:130–136, 1988.
17. Jones BJM, Lees R, Andrews J, et al: Comparison of an elemental and polymeric enteral diet in patients with normal gastrointestinal function. Gut 24:78–84, 1983.
18. Fischer JE, Funovics M, Aguirre A, et al: The role of plasma amino acids in hepatic encephalopathy. Surgery 78:276–290, 1975.
19. Rosen JM, Yoshimura N, Hodgman JM, Fischer JE: Plasma amino acid patterns in hepatic encephalopathy of differing etiology. Gastroenterology 72:483–487, 1977.

20. Naylor CD, O'Rourke K, Detsky AS, Baker JP: Parenteral nutrition with branched-chain amino acids in hepatic encephalopathy a meta-analysis. Gastro 97:1033–1042, 1989.
21. McGhee A, Henderson JM, Millikan WJ, et al: Comparison of the effects of Hepatic-Aid and a casein modular diet on encephalopathy, plasma amino acids, and nitrogen balance incirrhotic patients. Ann Surg 197:288–293, 1983.
22. Horst D, Grace ND, Conn HO, et al: Comparison of dietary protein with an oral, branched chain-enriched amino acid supplement in chronic portal-systemic encephalopathy: a randomized controlled trial. Hepatology 4:279–287, 1984.
23. Christie ML, Sack DM, Pomposelli J, Horst D: Enriched branched-chain amino acid formula versus a casein-based supplement in the treatment of cirrhosis. JPEN 9:671–678, 1985.
24. Egberts EH, Schomerus H, Hamster W, Jurgens P: Branched-chain amino acids in the treatment of latent portosystemic encephalopathy. Gastroenterology 88:887–895, 1985.
25. Bessman AN, Mitick GS, Hawkins R: Blood ammonia levels following the ingestion of casein and whole blood. J Clin Invest 37:990–998, 1958.
26. Fenton JCB, Knight EJ, Humpherson PL: Milk-and-cheese diet in portal-systemic encephalopathy. Lancet 1966:164–166.
27. Abel RM, Beck CH, Abbott WM, et al: Improved survival from acute renal failure after treatment with intravenous essential l-amino acids and glucose. Results of a prospective, double blind study. N Engl J Med 288:695–699, 1973.
28. Freund J, Atamian S, Fischer JE: Comparative study of parenteral nutrition in renal failure using essential and nonessential amino acid containing solutions. Surg Gynecol Obstet 151:652–656, 1980.
29. Varco R, Halliday D, Carson ER, et al: Efficiency of utilization of urea nitrogen for albumin synthesis by uremic and normal man. Clin Sci 48:379–390, 1975.
30. Feinstein EI, Blumenkrantz MJ, Healy M, et al: Clinical and metabolic responses to parenteral nutrition in acute renal failure: a controlled double-blind study. Medicine 60:124–137, 1981.
31. Mirtallo JM, Schneider PJ, Mavko K, et al: A comparison of essential and general amino acid infusions in the nutrition support of patients with compromised renal function. JPEN 6:109–113, 1982.
32. Stucki WP, Harper AE: Effects of altering the ratio of indispensable to dispensable amino acids in diets for rats. J Nutr 111:968–978, 1962.
33. Askanazi J, Elwyn DH, Silverberg PA, et al: Respiratory distress secondary to a high carbohydrate load: a case report. Surgery 87:596–598, 1980.
34. Askanazi J, Nordenstrom J, Rosenbaum SH, et al: Nutrition for the patient with respiratory failure: glucose vs. fat. Anesthesiology 54:373–377, 1981.
35. Serog P, Baigtes F, Apelfbaum M: Energy and nitrogen balance in 24 severely burned patients receiving four isocaloric diets of about 10MJ/m^2/day (2392 Kcalories/m^2/day). Burns 9:422–427, 1983.

36. Heymsfield SB, Head CA, McManus CB, et al: Respiratory, cardiovascular, and metabolic effects of enteral hyperalimentation: influence of formula dose and composition. Am J Clin Nutr 40:116–130, 1984.
37. Al-Saady NM, Blackmore CM, Bennett ED: High fat, low carbohydrate, enteral feeding lowers $PaCo_2$ and reduces the period of ventilation in artificially ventilated patients. Intensive Care Med 15:290–295, 1989.
38. Kane RE, Hobbs PJ, Black PG: Comparison of low, medium and high carbohydrate formulas for nighttime enteral feedings in cystic fibrosis patients. JPEN 14:47–52, 1990.
39. Mochizuki J, Trocki O, Dominioni L, et al: Optimal lipid content for enteral diets following thermal injury. JPEN 8:638–646, 1984.
40. Peters AL, Davidson MB, Isaac RM: Lack of glucose elevation after simulated tube feeding with a low-carbohydrate, high-fat enteral formula in patients with type I diabetes. Am J Med 87:178–182, 1989.
41. Bower RH, Muggia-Sullam M, Ballgren S, et al: Branched chain amino acid-enriched solutions in the septic patient: a randomized prospective trial. Ann Surg 203:13–20, 1986.
42. Cerra FB, Mazuski J, Teasley K, et al: Nitrogen retention in critically ill patients is proportional to the branched chain acid load. Crit Care Med 11:775–778, 1983.
43. Cerra FB, Mazuski J, Chute E, et al: Branched chain metabolic support: a prospective, randomized, double-blind trial in surgical stress. Ann Surg 199:286–291, 1984.
44. Cerra FB, Shronts EP, Konstantinides NN, et al: Enteral feeding in sepsis: a prospective, randomized, double-blind trial. Surgery 98:632–639, 1985.
45. Pelosi G, Proietti R, Magalini SI, et al: Anticatabolic properties of branched chain amino acids in trauma. Resuscitation 1983, 10:153–158.
46. Mochizuki H, Trocki O, Dominioni L, Alexander JW: Effect of a diet rich in branched chin amino acids on severely burned guinea pigs. J Trauma 26:1077–1085, 1986.
47. Guidelines for the Scientific Review of Enteral Food Products for Special Medical Purposes. Life Sciences Research Office, Federation of American Societies for Experimental Biology, December, 1990.
48. Brennan MF, Cerra F, Daly JM, et al: Report of a research workshop: branched-chain amino acids in stress and injury. JPEN 10:446–452, 1986.
49. Saito H, Trocki O, Wang S, et al: Metabolic and immune effects of dietary arginine supplementation after burn. Arch Surg 122:784–789, 1987.
50. Daly JM, Reynolds J, Thom A, et al: Immune and metabolic effects of arginine in the surgical patient. Ann Surg 208:512–523, 1988.
51. Gottschlich MM, Jenkins M, Warden GD, et al: Differential effects of three enteral dietary regimens on selected outcome variables in burn patients. JPEN 14:225–236, 1990.
52. Lieberman MD, Shou J, Torres AS, et al: Effects of nutrient substrates on immune function. Nutrition 6:88–91, 1990.

53. Daly JM, Lieberman M, Goldine J, et al: Enteral nutrition with supplemental arginine, RNA and omega-3 fatty acids: a prospective clinical trial. JPEN 15(Suppl), 1991.
54. Rees RGP, Cooper TM, Beetham R, et al: Influence of energy and nitrogen contents of enteral diets on nitrogen balance: a double blind prospective controlled clinical trial. Gut 30:123–129, 1989.
55. Twyman D, Young AB, Ott L, et al: High protein enteral feedings: a means of achieving positive nitrogen balance in head injured patients. JPEN 9:679–684, 1985.
56. Taper LJ, Milam RS, McCallister MS, et al: Mineral retention in young men consuming soy-fiber-augmented liquid-formula diets. Am J Clin Nutr 48:305–311, 1988.
57. Heymsfield SB, Roongspisuthipong C, Evert M, et al: Fiber supplementation of enteral formulas: effects on the bioavailability of major nutrients and gastrointestinal tolerance. JPEN 12:265–273, 1988.
58. Shinnick FL, Hess RL, Fischer MH, Marlett JA: Apparent nutrient absorption and upper gastrointestinal transit with fiber-containing enteral feedings. Am J Clin Nutr 49:471–475, 1989.
59. Dobb GJ, Towler SC: Diarrhea during enteral feeding in the critically ill: a comparison of feeds with and without fibre. Intensive Care Med 16:252–255, 1990.
60. Rolandelli RH, Koruda MJ, Settle RG, Rombeau JL: The effect of enteral feedings supplemented with pectin on the healing of caloric anastomoses in the rat. Surgry 99:703–706, 1986.
61. Frankenfield DC, Beyer PL: Soy-polysaccharide fiber: effect on diarrhea in tube-fed head-injured patients. Am J Clin Nutr 50:533–538, 1989.
62. Hart GK, Dobb GJ: Effect of a fecal bulking agent on diarrhea during enteral feeding the critically ill. JPEN 12:465–468, 1988.
63. Liebl BH, Fischer MH, VanCalcar SC, Marlett JA: Dietary fiber and long-term large bowel response in enterally nourished nonambulatory profoundly retarded youth. JPEN 14:371–375, 1990.
64. Shankardass K, Chuchmach S, Chelswick K, et al: Bowel function of long-term tube-fed patients consuming formulae with and without dietary fiber. JPEN 14:508–512, 1990.
65. Zimmaro DM, Rolandelli RH, Koruda MJ, et al: Isotonic tube feeding formula induces liquid stool in normal subjects: reversal by pectin. JPEN 13:117–123, 1989.
66. Palacio JC, Rombeau JL: Dietary fiber: a brief review and potential application to enteral nutrition. Nutr Clin Pract 5:99–106, 1990.
67. Scheppach W, Burghardt W, Bartram P, Kasper H: Addition of dietary fiber to liquid formula diets: the pros and cons. JPEN 14:204–209, 1990.
68. Silk DBA: Fibre and enteral nutrition. Gut 30:246–264, 1989.
69. Edes TE, Walk BE, Austin JL: Diarrhea in tube-fed patients: feeding formula not necessarily the cause. Am J Med 88:91–93, 1990.

70. Gottschlich MM, Warden GD, Michel MA, et al: Diarrhea in tube-fed burn patients: incidence, etiology, nutritional impact, and prevention. JPEN 12:338–345, 1988.
71. Viall C, Porcelli K, Teran JC, et al: A double-blind clinical trial comparing the gastrointestinal side effects of two enteral feeding formulas. JPEN 14:265–269, 1990.
72. Ford EG, Jennings LM, Andrassy RJ: Serum albumin (oncotic pressure) correlates with enteral feeding tolerance in the pediatric surgical patient. Pediatr Surg 22:597–599, 1987.
73. Patterson ML: Enteral feeding in the hypoalbuminemic patient. JPEN 14(4):362–365.
74. Keohane PP, Attrill H, Love M, et al: Relation between osmolality of diet and gastrointestinal side effects in enteral nutrition. Br Med J 288:678–680, 1984.
75. Zarling EJ, Parmar JR, Mobarhan S, Clapper M: Effect of enteral formula infusion rate, osmolality and chemical composition upon clinical tolerance and carbohydrate absorption in normal subjects. JPEN 10:588–590, 1986.

CHAPTER 11

Early Enteral Feeding Via a Jejunostomy: A Safe Technique in Critically Ill Patients

*Thomas L. Khoury, M.D.,
Bradley C. Borlase, M.D., M.S.,
R. Armour Forse, M.D., Ph.D.,
Stacey J. Bell, M.S., R.D., CNSD,
Wendy Swails, R.D., CNSD,
George L. Blackburn, M.D., Ph.D.,
and Bruce R. Bistrian, M.D., Ph.D.*

There is a growing interest in using enteral nutrition to support critically ill patients in the immediate postoperative period. Randomized studies have shown improved outcome, decreased lengths of stay (particularly when specialized enteral diets are used) (1), and reduced cost (2) in patients receiving enteral nutrition compared to parenteral nutrition. What remains controversial is the preferred route of enteral access: nasal intubation vs. percutaneous placement guided by an endoscope versus surgical placement. Use of stomach in the critically ill patient is hindered by the high likelihood of problems from delayed gastric emptying, leading to vomiting and the potential for pulmonary aspiration. Our hospital has a significant subset (30%) of diabetic patients and, when combined with critical illness, their condition could result in a high degree of intolerance to enteral feeding given intragastrically (3). Feeding jejunostomies may bypass the problem of feeding intolerances seen with gastric feedings. However, they

Note: The authors gratefully acknowledge Kathleen Dascoulias, DTR, for her technical support and Tracey Doyle for her expert word processing work on the manuscript.

reportedly have a high complication rate in terms of tolerance to the enteral diet and surgical placement of the tube (4–6).

Due to this reportedly high complication rate and the published reports of bowel ischemia associated with jejunostomy feedings (5), we prospectively collected data on all patients with a surgically placed feeding jejunostomy, with emphasis on the associated complications, for 1 year.

METHODS

All consecutive patients in 1990 who were fed postoperatively (within 12 hr) via a surgically placed jejunostomy tube were included in the study. Demographic parameters, nutritional indices, comorbid diseases, admission source and service, outcome, and complications were reviewed. Feeding tube placement in relationship to the anastomosis, if present, as well as the type of tube and enteral formula, and patient outcome were also described.

Patients with nasojejunal tubes were not included in this study. A subset of these (n = 14) had diagnoses of Crohn's disease, inflammatory bowel disease, or ascites, which represented contraindications for surgical placement of jejunostomy feeding tubes.

Patients were evaluated for one minor complication: diarrhea (defined as more than three stools daily). Several major catheter-related (catheter-dislodgement and bowel ischemia) and non-catheter-related complications were assessed: septicemia, positive blood culture, intra-abdominal abscess, fistula, urinary tract infection, pneumonia, wound infection, wound dehiscence, small bowel obstruction, and shock.

Criteria for these complications were adapted from Mullen et al. (7). Septicemia required at least one positive blood culture associated with hypotension (defined by a systolic blood pressure <90 mmHg) and hypoperfusion. Intra-abdominal sepsis was defined as an intra-abdominal purulent collection requiring operative or radiologic drainage. Fistulas were documented radiographically. A diagnosis of a urinary tract infection required a quantitative urine culture of greater than 100,000 organisms. Pneumonia was documented by an abnormal chest x-ray, positive sputum culture, and treatment with antibiotics. The presence of a wound infection required documentation by culture and operative or spontaneous drainage of purulent material. Wound dehiscence required operative reclosure of the wound. Small bowel obstruction was confirmed by clinical signs and x-rays. A diagnosis of shock required hypotension, hypoperfusion, and treatment with systemic vasopressor. A diagnosis of bowel ischemia was made at reexploration.

TABLE 11-1. Patient Characteristics (n=51)

	Patients	
	n	%
Gender		
Males	32	64
Admitting service		
Cardiothoracic	13	25
General surgery	31	60
Transplantation	5	10
Head and neck	2	5
Admission source		
Elective	25	50
Acute transfers	13	25
Emergency room	13	25
Patient outcome		
Discharged	48	94
Died	3	6
Discharge home with tube (n=19)		
Receiving tube feeding diet	14	74 (subgroup of 19)
Use tube for hydration	1	5
Tube clamped, not removed	4	21

RESULTS

Fifty-one consecutive patients with jejunal feeding catheters were reviewed. Forty-two (82%) of the feeding jejunostomies were placed at the time of the patient's primary operation. The average age of patients was 63 years, with 60% of the patients admitted to the general surgery service (Table 11-1) followed by the cardiothoracic service, which admitted 25%. Half of the patients were admitted electively and the remaining half included equal numbers of acute transfer and emergency room cases.

There were three (6%) deaths, all from multiple system organ failure, unrelated to the feeding tube. Of the remaining 48 patients, 40% (19) were discharged with their feeding tube. Fourteen of these received a tube feeding formula, one received hydration via the tube, and four had the tubes clamped. The remaining 29 patients demonstrated the ability to adequately hydrate (consume at least 1 L of fluid per day) and nourish (consume at least 1,000 kCal per day) themselves orally at an adequate level. Therefore, their feeding tubes were removed before they were discharged.

Nutritional indices revealed a mild to moderately malnourished population

TABLE 11-2. Nutritional Assessment

Parameter	Value	Degree of Malnutrition
Serum albumin (g/dl)	3.0 ± 0.7	Moderate
Total lymphocyte count (cells/mm^3)	1320 ± 710	Mild
≥ 10% weight change	21%	Severe

Values given as mean ± standard deviation.

TABLE 11-3. Comorbidity in 51 Patients with a Feeding Jejunostomy

Comorbid Condition	Patients n	Patients %	Comments
Diabetes mellitus	18	35	Type I and type II
Renal insufficiency	8	16	Patients receiving and/or dialysis creatinine>2
Cardiac disease	8	16	History of CAD and/or a CABG
Vascular disease	5	10	Peripheral vascular disease with a history of claudication and/or bypass surgery
None	12	23	

(Table 11-2). The mean admission serum albumin concentration was 3.0 g/dl and total lymphocyte count was 1320 cell/mm^3 which represented moderate and mild malnourishment, respectively. One-fifth of patients had experienced a severe weight loss prior to admission (≥ 10% usual body weight).

There was a significant subset (77%) of patients with comorbid disease (Table 11-3). Thirty-five percent of patients were diabetic, 16% had renal insufficiency, 10% had vascular disease, and 16% had a history of coronary artery disease.

Three patients (6%) experienced catheter dislodgement, which was considered to be a major complication since the catheters were placed solely for feeding purposes (Table 11-4). In two patients the tube fell out; one occurred 2 days after insertion and the other 11 days after insertion. Both of these patients had their jejunostomies placed as secondary procedures. The third patient complained of abdominal pain when the tube feeding diet was initiated. The patient's tube was placed as a primary procedure following an esophagogastrectomy several months earlier. He was investigated radiologically and the tube was identified lying freely in the peritoneal activity. Although the exact reason for dislodgement could not be determined, the patient did not develop peritonitis, and a new tube was easily inserted in the same tract.

The only other major complication occurred in a 75-year-old patient who had undergone an aortic valve and mitral heart valve replacement and required prolonged ventilator support postoperatively (Table 11-4). In the immediate

TABLE 11-4. Complications (n=51)

Complications	Patients n	%
Major		
Catheter-related		
Catheter dislodgment		
Intraperitoneal	1	2
Out of wound	2	4
Ischemic bowel	1	2
Non-catheter-related		
Positive blood culture	9	18
Wound infection	9	18
Septicemia	6	12
Urinary tract infection	6	12
Pneumonia	3	6
Intra-abdominal abscess	2	4
Fistula	1	2
Wound dehiscence	1	2
Minor (Non-catheter-related)		
Diarrhea	3	6

postoperative period, the patient was nutritionally and metabolically supported with parenteral nutrition. Three weeks later, a tracheostomy was placed, and enteral feedings were initiated via an endoscopically placed postpyloric feeding tube. This tube was inadvertently pulled back and the tip became lodged in the stomach. Subsequent attempts to feed this patient nasogastrically were unsuccessful as demonstrated by persistently high gastric residuals. Thus, in conjunction with the rewiring of her sternum for dehiscence, a feeding jejunostomy was placed via an abdominal incision.

During this procedure, the patient became hypotensive (blood pressure 90–95 mmHg) for 15–15 min, but no obvious ill effects were noted at the time of operation. A full-strength polymeric tube feeding diet was administered via the feeding jejunostomy at 10 ml/hr in the recovery room. The following day, the administration rate of the formula was increased to 30 ml/hr. A fever and abdominal distention were noted on postoperative day 2. A radiographic study of the feeding tube revealed no intraperitoneal leak. However, due to a deteriorating clinical condition, she was re-explored on postoperative day 3 and found to have a necrotic cecum distended at 13 cm and patchy ischemic necrosis of her transverse and descending colon. The site of the feeding jejunostomy showed no signs of ischemia. The patient subsequently underwent resection of the right colon. Enteral feeds were restarted at 10 ml/hr via the original feeding jejunostomy, in the

TABLE 11-5. Relationship of Tube to Anastomosis (n=51)

Location	n	%
Above anastomosis	13	25
Below anastomosis	15	30
No anastomosis	23	45

recovery room. An elemental formula (low in fat and consisting of protein as free amino acids) rather than a polymeric formula (higher in fat and containing intact protein) was used at this time. Parenteral nutrition provided most of the calories during the early postoperative period as the enteral feeding rate was slowly being advanced. By postoperative day 5, the enteral feeding reached goal rate, and the intravenous nutrition was discontinued. The patient was eventually discharged, and was alive and well 10 months later.

The most prevalent major, non-catheter-related complications were an 18% (n=9) incidence of a positive blood culture, which was directly related to intravascular monitoring devices and central access for parenteral fluids, and wound infection (18%) (Table 11-4). This was followed by septicemia (12%), urinary tract infection (12%), pneumonia (6%), intra-abdominal abscess (4%), fistula (2%), and wound dehiscence (2%). The fistulas were not directly related to the feeding jejunostomy, and no small bowel obstructions or incidences of shock occurred.

The sole minor, non-catheter-related complication monitored was diarrhea. Six percent of patients (n=3) exhibited diarrhea.

All patients who were re-explored after placement of a feeding jejunostomy during a previous surgery had their catheters left in place except one. This patient had severe protein–calorie malnutrition and wound dehiscence of his surgical incision. After the patient showed no signs of healing, the catheter was prophylactically removed because of the fear of leakage.

Twenty-eight patients had small bowel anastomoses; 13 (25%) were fed above and 15 (30%) below (Table 11-5). Twenty-three (45%) patients had no anastomosis.

Most patients (76%) received large (> 10 Fr.) feeding tubes placed by the Witzel technique (Table 11-6). Fourteen percent received needle catheter jejunostomies and the remainder had T-tubes fashioned as described by Maingot and inserted into the jejunum (8).

Most (83%) of the patients received one of the two different elemental formulas in the early postoperative period. Both diets were low in fat (<10% of the total calories) and had protein in the form of free amino acids (FAA) or FAA and small peptides. The remaining patients received a variety of polymeric formulas containing approximately 30% fat and intact protein.

TABLE 11-6. Type of Tube and Formula Used in the Early Postoperative Period (n=51)

	Patients	
	n	%
Tubes		
Red rubber tube: Witzel method (10–14 Fr)	39	76
Needle catheter	7	14
T-tube (12–14 Fr)	5	10
Formulas		
Elemental		
Vital HN[a]	31	56
Vivonex TEN[b]	15	27
Polymeric		
Osmolite[a]	6	11
Sustacal[c]	1	2
Ensure[a]	1	2
Impact[d]	1	2

[a]Ross Laboratory (Columbia OH).
[b]Norwich Eaton (Norwich, NY).
[c]Mead Johnson (Evansville, IN).
[d]Sandoz Nutrition (Minneapolis, MN).

DISCUSSION

Enteral nutrition has recently become an increasingly popular means of alimenting the critically ill, hospitalized patient due to its theoretic advantages in terms of immunity and metabolism. Moreover, it is less costly than parenteral feeding. We have described a series of 51 consecutive patients who were fed by surgically placed jejunostomy tubes, usually in conjunction with total parenteral nutrition (TPN) and converted gradually to total enteral feeding. There were 3 (6%) incidences of catheter dislodgement, which was considered a major complication. There was also one major complication: a patient developed ischemic bowel. This patient was clearly at risk for decreased mesenteric blood flow given her poor cardiac status. However, it remains unclear whether this event was precipitated by her poor vascular status, her hypotensive event in the operating room, the initiation of enteral feeding, or a combination of these factors.

The non-jejunostomy-related major complications were typically found in surgical patients. The most common problems were a positive blood culture associated with the need for parenteral access, and wound infection at the site of the surgical incision.

In another reported study (5), the placement and use of feeding jejunostomies has been associated with an overall 55% complication rate, of which 9% (4% life-threatening, 5% mortality) were major complications. The authors attribute these rates to ischemic complications. Patients with risk factors for diminished mesenteric blood flow are at increased risk for ischemic bowel. Complications in the aforementioned study were reported without reference to the tube used. Moreover, the authors of the above study noted a moderate success rate with enteral feeding. These authors observed a much higher incidence of diarrhea (29% vs. 6%) than we did. However, it is certainly worth noting that their initial infusion rates were two and a half times higher than our modest initial rate of 10 ml/hr.

Hayashi et al. (6) found relatively poor success using a catheter jejunostomy in patients who had undergone upper abdominal surgery. Despite the fact that all patients (n=11) received elemental diets (Vivonex HN, Norwich Eaton; or Criticare HN, Mead Johnson, 65% of the patients experienced gastrointestinal discomfort leading to cessation or curtailment of tube feeding. The complications included diarrhea, abdominal pain and distension, and retrograde reflex of feeding into the stomach. We avoided most of these problems, and thus the curtailment of feeding, because of our slow initiation rate and modest calorie goal. These authors (6) began feeding at 45 ml/hr on day 1 postoperatively and provided up to 3000 kCal/day as the final goal. Our patients rarely received more than 2000 kCal daily. In 1985, when the study (6) was published this was the acceptable caloric goal but today goals are more modest (9).

Although Hayashi et al. (6) found no postoperative mortality, 1 of 11 patients experienced a placement complication, which could be considered a major complication: an abscess formed in the abdominal wall, which required drainage several days after removal of the catheter. Moreover, 2 of 11 patients had anastomic leaks, of which we had none.

In contrast, we had 100% success with our formula administration using a feeding technique that begins feedings in the first 6–12 hr following surgical placement of the feeding tube (see Figure 17-1), usually in the recovery room, with a full-strength elemental diet administered at 10 ml/hr. We have previously demonstrated high tolerance rates with a low incidence of diarrhea (10). Patients are usually fully nutritionally supported by the enteral route by day 4 or 5, and most patients are able to undergo the transition to a polymeric formula before discharge.

Many physicians are concerned about intraluminal gastrointestinal feeding when an anastomosis is present. This is a serious concern, but if the proper feeding techniques are used, there is little danger of leak due to the feedings. When feedings are started at 10 ml/hr for the first 24 hr, this allows the preservation of mucosal integrity while providing only 240 ml of extra gastrointestinal volume.

It is important to note that the gastrointestinal tract will routinely pass 1–2 L of bowel contents through an anastomosis daily in a fasted state. In view of this, anastomotic leakage is always due to poor surgical technique not enteral feeding.

Diarrhea not associated with *C. difficile* can be a major associated complication of enteral feedings (3). However, it is more likely to be associated with antibiotic use and/or medications containing sorbitol, a compound as effective as lactulose in treating constipation (11). The incidence of diarrhea in this study was 6%, and in our previous prospectively randomized trial in patients with mean serum albumin concentrations of 2.3 g/dl, the rate was 10–15% (10) in both groups, representing a very acceptable incidence rate.

Enteral feeding increases gastrointestinal blood flow from approximately 5% of the cardiac output to 15% (12). In patients with significant vascular disease and/or associated diabetes, it is always of great concern that aggressive enteral feeding may cause ischemic bowel in the early postoperative period. In this study, we describe a patient who was fed during the early postoperative period with a standard jejunal feeding tube and later developed an ischemic right colon that required resection. The patient was successfully fed enterally after the colonic resection with no further gastrointestinal problems. A cause-and-effect relationship is not implied from this case, but it may identify a select subset of patients in whom enteral feeding must be done very conservatively.

In summary, a review of 51 surgical patients with 52 feeding jejunostomies was carried out. Three (6%) patients experienced catheter dislodgement, one requiring reoperation for replacement, and one major complication of colonic infarction occurred in a patient who had a hypotensive period during surgery. There were three (6%) deaths unrelated to the feeding tube. Feeding jejunostomies can be a cost-effective therapy with an excellent risk–benefit ratio for the critically ill patient undergoing major theracoabdominal surgery. Complications can be minimized by using good surgical technique, paying close attention to the patient's hemodynamic status, monitoring gastrointestinal symptoms such as abdominal distention, and giving careful consideration to feeding rate and formula type.

REFERENCES

1. Daly JM, Lieberman M, Goldfine J, Shou J, Weintraub FW, Rosato EF, Lavin P: Enteral nutrition with supplemental arginine, RNA and omega-3 fatty acids: a prospective clinical trial. Surgery 1992.
2. Bower RH, Talamini MA, Sax HC, Hamilton F, Fischer JE: Postoperative enteral vs parenteral nutrition. Arch Surg 121:1040–1045 (1986).
3. Borlase BC, Babineau TJ, Forse RA, Bell SJ, Blackburn GL: Enteral nutrition support. In: Rippe JM, Irwin RS, Alpert JS, Fink MP: Intensive Care Medicine, 2nd edition. Boston: Little, Brown, 1992.

4. Daly JM, Bonau R, Stofberg P, Bloch A, Jeevanandam M, Morse M: Immediate postoperative jejunostomy feeding. Am J Surg 153:198–206, 1987.
5. Smith-Choban P, Max MH: Feeding jejunostomy: a small bowel streess test. Am J Surg 155:112–117, 1988.
6. Hayashi JT, Wolfe BM, Calvert EC. Limited efficacy of early postoperative jejunal feeding. Am J Surg 150:52–57, 1985.
7. Mullen JL, Buzby GP, et al: Reduction of operative morbidity and mortality by combined preoperative and postoperative nutritional support. Ann Surg 192(5):604–613 (1980).
8. Ellis H. Choledocholithiasis, in Norwalk, CT: Maingot's Abdominal Operations, Schwartz SI, Ellis H (eds). Appleton-Century Crofts, 1985, p. 1900.
9. Hunter DC, Jaskic T, Lewis D, Bistrian BR, Blackburn GL: Resting energy expenditure in the critically ill: estimations versus measurement. Br J Surg 75:875–878, 1988.
10. Borlase BC, Bell SJ, Lewis EJ, Swails W, Bistrian BR, Forse RA, Blackburn GL: Tolerance to enteral tube feeding diets in hypoalbuminemic critically ill, geriatric patients: a prospective randomized trial. Surg Gynecol Obstet 174:181–188, 1992.
11. Edes TE, Walk BE, Austin JL: Diarrhea in tube-fed patients: feeding formula not necessarily the cause. Am J Med 88:91–93, 1990.
12. Guyton AC: in Guyton AC (ed) Textbook of Medical Physiology. Philadelphia: WB Saunders, 1981, p. 350.

PRACTICAL APPLICATIONS FOR ENTERAL NUTRITION

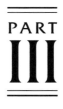

PART III

Who Should Receive Enteral Nutrition and What Are the Nutrient Requirements?

CHAPTER 12

Martha Lebow, R.D., CNSD

PATIENT CRITERIA FOR ENTERAL NUTRITION USAGE

Based on the American Society of Enteral and Parenteral Nutrition (ASPEN) Guidelines for Enteral Feeding (1), the following clinical situations warrant administration of enteral nutrition.

In the following clinical settings, enteral nutrition should be a part of routine care.

- Protein–calorie malnutrition (> 10% loss of usual weight or serum albumin levels < 3.5 g/dl) with inadequate intake of nutrients for the previous 5 days
- Normal nutritional status with less than 50% of required nutrient intake orally for the previous 7–10 days
- Severe dysphagia
- Major full-thickness burns
- Small bowel resection in combination with administration of total parenteral nutrition (TPN)

In the following clinical settings, enteral nutrition would usually be helpful.

Major trauma (enteral nutrition would be contraindicted if paralytic ileus ensues)
Radiation therapy
Mild chemotherapy
Liver failure and severe renal dysfunction

In the following clinical settings, enteral nutrition is of limited or undetermined value.

Intensive chemotherapy (parenteral nutrition may be indicated for individuals with severe symptoms)
Immediate postoperative period if patient is expected to resume oral intake with 5–7 days
Acute enteritis
Less than 10% small intestine remaining

Enteral nutrition should not be used in the following clinical settings.

Complete mechanical intestinal obstruction
Ileus or intestinal hypomotility
Severe diarrhea (resistance to pharmacologic therapy)
High-output external fistulas (>500 ml/day)
Severe acute pancreatitis
Patients with hypovolemic or septic shock
Not desired by the patient or legal guardian
Prognosis does not warrant aggressive nutritional support.

MACRONUTRIENT REQUIREMENTS

These are summarized in Table 12-1 and described below.

Caloric Requirements

Before the routine use of indirect calorimetry for patient care units in many hospitals across the country, clinicians assumed that critically ill patients were extremely hypermetabolic and required more than twice their predicted metabolic rate in calories. We now know that their needs are much less and often only slightly in excess of normal basal energy expenditure (BEE) (approximately 20 kCal/kg body weight). A more accurate way to determine BEE is by use of the

Harris-Benedict Equations, which are multiple linear regression equations using selected characteristics of the patient's age, gender, height, and weight (2):

REE for female = 66.4230 + 13.7516W + 5.0033H − 3.7750A
REE for male = 655.0955 + 9.6534W + 1.8496H − 4.6756A

where A is age in years, H is height in centimeters, W is weight in kilograms, and REE is resting energy expenditure in kCal per day.

These equations have recently come under scrutiny, particularly in malnourished patients who may either be markedly cachetic or have exaggerated body weight due to edema or ascites. Use of urinary creatinine levels has been proposed as an alternative (3).

Most patients exhibit some degree of hypermetabolism over basal needs and Hunter et al. have summarized energy needs as follows: Thirty kCal/kg will give sufficient calories for 90% of patients, but 20% would receive an excess of 1000 kCal/day, 15% would be fed double their needs, and 30 kCal/kg would only be advocated for nonventilated patients and for patients in whom excessive intake is not of major concern (e.g., patients who would not be harmed by overfeeding by a moderate amount: unstressed, malnourished patients with otherwise good organ function such as those with anorexia nervosa.

In sum, our caloric goals are, for patients in the intensive care unit (ICU), 20–25 kCal/kg actual body weight; and for those not in the intensive care unit, 30 kCal/kg actual body weight.

Protein

Unlike caloric needs, protein requirements of the critically ill approximate twice the normal needs of 0.8/kg body weight. This is needed to compensate for increased stress, activated immune system, excess nitrogen losses, and repletion of body stores. Based on results of nitrogen balance studies and more sophisticated protein kinetic modeling, the most severely stressed patients (major burns) may require at most 2.5 g protein/kg (three times the recommended daily allowance [RDA]). Patients in the ICU and non-ICU setting should receive 1.5 g protein/kg (3). As the degree of stress abates, nitrogen loss is less and intake may be reduced to 1.0–1.2 g protein/kg prior to discharge.

Underfeeding of protein to patients with nitrogen retention disorders (primarily due to hepatic or renal insufficiency) is not a reasonable approach to the problem; treatment of the disease is the only permanent solution. These patients have the same protein needs as other hospitalized patients, and if they are not met exogenously, the body will catabolize its own protein-rich stores, first in the muscle and then in vital organs. In order to ameliorate nitrogen (as blood urea

TABLE 12-1. Estimation of Macronutrient Requirements

Macronutrient	Non-ICU Patient 1	ICU Patients 2	Exceptions	70 kg patient; 1: Non-ICU 2: ICU
kCal	25–30 kCal/kg ABW	20–25 kCal/kg ABW	Obese: use midway between ABW and IBW	1: 30 × 70 = 2100 kCal 2: 22 × 70 = 1540 kCal
Protein	1.2–1.5 g/kg/IBW	1.5 g/kg/IBW	Nitrogen retention disorder: use BCAA-enriched formula and provide 1.0 g/kg/IBW	1: 1.2 × 70 = 84 g 2: 1.5 × 70 = 105 g
CHO	2.5–4.0 mg/kg/min ABW	2.5–4.0 mg/kg/min ABW	Obese: use midway between ABW and IBW	252–403 g
Fat	Remaining kCals	Remaining kCals	If ventilator-dependent and intragastrically fed, should receive <10% kCal as fat	Total kCal − [protein kCal + cholesterol] = fat kCal 1: 2100 − [(84 g protein × 4 kCal/g) + (350 g cholesterol × 4 kCal/g)] = 2100 kCal−(336+1400) = 364 kCal = 40 g fat 2: 1540 − [105 g protein × 4 kCal/g) + (252 g cholesterol × 4 kCal/g)] = 1540−(420+1008) = 112 kCal = 12 g fat
Total fluid needs	30 cc/kg	30 cc/kg	Fluid retention: follow in & out	70 × 30 = 2100 ml

ABW, actual body weight; IBW, ideal body weight

nitrogen [BUN] or NH_3) build-up in the blood, administration of protein sources, enriched with the branched chain amino acids (BCAAs) (leucine, isoleucine, and valine) to a final concentration of 40–50%, has been advocated. BCAA-enriched diets have been shown to enhance protein synthesis while minimizing catabolism (4). For enterally fed patients, we suggest use of BCAA-enriched formulas with roughly half the protein comprised of the BCAAs. Because these proteins are more efficiently utilized, less is required (1.0 g/kg). After the medical problem causing the nitrogenous build-up is corrected, patients should return to being fed with the standard protein source because they are better for whole body protein synthesis and far less costly.

In sum, protein needs for patients in the ICU are 1.5 g protein/kg; for nonstressed/stable patients, 1.0–1.2 g protein/kg; and for those with nitrogen retention disorder, 1.0 g protein enriched with BCAA/kg.

Carbohydrate

Carbohydrate serves as the primary source of energy for the brain, red blood cell, and soft tissues. In a nonstressed state, when a suboptimal amount of carbohydrate is given, gluconeogenesis will occur via the catabolism of protein and thus should be avoided. When excess carbohydrate is provided, it is converted to triglycerides which are often stored in the liver. Continuous overfeeding of carbohydrate to an immobilized patient results in an increased respiratory quotient (RQ) (CO_2 expired air/O_2 consumed). CO_2 production becomes elevated from the synthesis of triglycerides from glucose. Glucose intakes between 2.5 and 4.0 mg/kg/min have been shown to suppress gluconeogenesis while keeping the RQ < 1, which is a desirable range for ventilated-dependent patients who are about to be extubated, or for ventilator-dependent patients who have difficulty ridding the body of CO_2 (e.g., those with chronic obstructive pulmonary disease) (5).

Fat

Fat is the most calorically dense source of nutrients and is required to prevent essential fatty acid deficiency. However, only 4% of calories need to come from a vegetable oil rich in the essential fatty acid linoleic acid to satisfy these requirements. Recent investigations have identified deleterious side effects, particularly in the immune system, from overfeeding omega-6 (from vegetable oils primarily). Recently developed fats, such as medium-chain triglycerides (MCTs) that are readily oxidized and unable to be stored, are excellent alternatives (6). Fish oils (rich in omega-3 fatty acids) actually dampen the immune response and may be preferred to the omega-6 group during periods of inflammation (7).

REFERENCES

1. ASPEN Board of Directors: Guidelines for the use of enteral nutrition in the adult patient. JPEN 5:435–439, 1987.
2. Hunter DC, Jaksic T, Lewis D, Benotti PN, Blackburn GL, Bistrian BR: Resting energy expenditure in the critically ill: estimation vs. measurement. Br J Surg 75:875–878, 1988.
3. Chwals W, Blackburn GL: Perioperative nutritional support in the cancer patient. Surg Clin North Am 66:1137–1165, 1986.
4. Shanbhogue LKR, Bistrian BR, Swensen S, Blackburn GL: Twenty-four hour urinary creatinine: a simple technique for estimating resting energy expenditure in normal population and the hospitalized patients. Clin Nutr 6:221–225, 1987.
5. Shanbhogue LKR, Chwals WJ, Weintraub M, Blackburn GL, Bistrian BR: Parenteral nutrition in the surgical patient. Br J Surg 74:172–180, 1987.
6. Burke JF, Wolfe RR, Mullany CJ, Matthews DE, Bier DM: Glucose requirements following burn injury. Ann Surg 190:274–285, 1979.
7. Bach AC, Babayan VK: Medium-chain triglycerides: an update. Am J Clin Nutr 36:950–962, 1982.
8. Pomposelli JJ, Mascioli EA, Bistrian BR, Lopes SM, Blackburn GL: Attenuation of the febrile response in guinea pigs by fish oil enriched diets. JPEN Nutr 13:136–140, 1989.

Micronutrient Additives

CHAPTER 13

Wendy Swails, R.D., CNSD

Enteral formulas contain sufficient electrolytes and vitamins and minerals to meet most patients' needs. Most formulas have 100% of the United States recommended daily allowances (RDAs) in 1200–2000 ml. The RDAs were established to meet the needs of a normal, healthy population, and thus may be insufficient for a hospitalized population. Thus, supplementation with selected nutrients may be required for certain patients. Selected vitamin and mineral additives are presented in Table 13-1.

Enteral formulas contain modest amounts of sodium and potassium (20–35 mEq/L each). This amount is usually sufficient to meet patients' needs, yet more is sometimes required. The need for sodium and potassium varies among disease states, especially in depleted patients, those in renal and hepatic failure, and in stressed patients with large third space. Available additives are presented in Table 13-2. If sodium and/or potassium present in the enteral formula is contraindicated (*e.g.*, in patients with hepatic and/or renal failure), Hepatic-Aid II (McGaw) is nearly free of these electrolytes (and virtually all vitamins and minerals). Although designed for patients with hepatic failure, it can be used for those with hepatic and renal failure. Calculation of the additive needed must be as specific as possible.

TABLE 13-1. Vitamin/Mineral and Electrolyte Preparations

Additive	Chemical	Form	Elemental	RDA	Dosage	Cost ($)
VITAMINS						
Vitamin A						
Aquasol A		Softgel capsule 7.5 mg	7500 μg retinol (25,000 IU)	800–1000 μg (2664–3330 IU)	Xerophthalmia: 500,000 IU/day × 3 days, followed by 50,000 IU/day × 2 weeks	0.83/7.5 mg 1.45/15 mg
		15 mg	15,000 μg retinol (50,000 IU)		Severe deficiency: 100,000 IU/day × 3 days, followed by 50,000 IU/day × 2 weeks	
					Follow up: 10,000–20,000 IU/day × 2 mths	
Vitamin B1 (Thiamin)						
Thiamine hydrochloride	Thiamine HCL	IM, IV 2 ml vial	100 mg/ml	1.0–1.5 mg	Beriberi: 10–20 mg/IV 3 x/day × 2wks	0.95/ml
					Wernicke-Korsakoff: 100 mg IV initially; 50–100 mg/day IM maintenance until consuming adequate POs	
Vitamin B1		Crushable tablets	50 mg 100 mg	1.0–1.5 mg	Daily supplement: 5–30 mg orally/day	0.08/50 or 100 mg

Vitamin B6 (Pyridoxine)					
Hexa-Betalin	Pyridoxine hydrochloride	IM 10 ml vial	100 mg/ml	1.6–2.0 mg	Dietary deficiency: 10–20 mg/day × 3 weeks, followed by oral MVI containing 2–5 mg vitamin B6	22.70/10 ml
					Vitamin B6 dependency syndrome: 30 mg/day for life
Vitamin B6	Crushable tablets		50 mg 100 mg	1.6–2.0 mg		0.08/50 or 100 mg
Vitamin B12 (Cobalamin)					
Cyanocobalamin		IM, SC 1 ml vial	100 μ/ml 1000 μg/ml	2.0 μg	Pernicious anemia: 100 μg × 6–7 days; if reticulocyte count improved, 100 μg daily × 7 days; then 100 μg q 3–4 days × 2–3 wks; then 100 μg/month for life	1.70/100 μg 0.91/1000 μg
Vitamin B12		Tablet	50 μg 250 μg	20 μg		0.04/50 μg tablet 0.08/250 μg tablet
Vitamin E (Tocopheryl)					
Vitamin E		Soft gel capsule	100 IU 400 IU 1000 IU	8–10 mg (12–15 IU)		0.12/100 IU 0.17/400 IU 0.46/1000 IU
Vitamin K					
Phytonadione		Tablet	5 mg	60–80 μg		1.62/tablet
Vitamin K		IV 1 ml vial	10 mg/ml	60–80 μg		13.28 ml

TABLE 13-1. (Continued)

Additive	Chemical	Form	Elemental	RDA	Dosage	Cost ($)
VITAMINS—continued						
Niacin						
Niacin		Crushable tablet	50 mg 100 mg	13–19 mg	Niacin deficiency: 10–20 mg daily Pellagra: up to 500 mg/day	0.08/50 or 100 mg
MINERALS						
Calcium						
Calcium chloride	$CaCl_2$	IV 10% 10 ml vial (1 g $CaCL_2$)	270 mg (13.6 mEq) Ca/10 ml	800–1200 mg (40–60 mEq)	5–10 ml q 1–3 days	1.37/10 ml
Calcium gluconate		IV 10% 10 ml vial	90 mg (4.5 mEq) Ca/ml	800–1200 mg	500–2000 mg (5–20 ml)	1.33/10 ml
Calcium gluconate		Crushable tablets 500 mg 1g	45 mg (2.3 mEq) Ca/500 mg 90 mg (4.5 mEq) Ca/1 g	800–1200 mg	1–4 tablets 3 times/day	0.21/500 mg or 1g
Calcium carbonate (Tums)	$CaCO_3$	Film-coated tablet 1250 mg	500 mg (25 mEq) Ca/tablet	800–1200 mg	1 tablet 2–3 times/day	0.17/tablet

Neo-calglucon	Syrup 30 ml	115 mg (5.8 mEq) Ca/5 ml	800–1200 mg	1 Tbls. (14.8 ml) 3 times/day	5.64/30 ml
Folic Acid					
Folic acid	IM, IV or SC 10 ml vial	5 mg folic acid/ml	180–200 μg	Therapeutic: up to 1 mg/day Maintenance: 0.4 mg/day	0.42/0.2 ml
Folic Acid	Tablet	1 mg folic acid/tablet	180–200 μg		0.08/tablet
Iron					
Imferon	IV, IM 2 ml vial	50 mg Fe/ml	10–15 mg	<2.0 ml/day Iron-deficiency anemia: 2 ml 0.0476 × wt (kg) × (nor hemoglobin observed hemoglobin) + 1 ml/5 kg (max. 14 ml)	42.00/
Ferrous sulfate	Elixir 300 mg FeSO$_4$/5 ml	60 mg Fe/5ml	10–15 mg	100–200 mg (2–3 mg/kg) elemental Fe/day in 3 divided doses	0.05/5 ml
Ferrous sulfate	FeSO$_4$ Enteric-coated tablet 325 mg	65 mg Fe/tablet	10–15 mg		0.08/tablet
Ferrous gluconate	Enteric-coated tablet 325 mg	38 mg Fe/tablet	10–15 mg		0.08/tablet
Ferrous gluconate	Elixir 300 mg/5 ml	35 mg Fe/5 ml	10–15 mg		0.42/5 ml
Magnesium					
Magnesium gluconate	Tablet 500 mg	27 mg (2.3 mEq) Mg/tablet	280–350 mg (23.3–29.2 mEq)		0.21/tablet

TABLE 13-1. (*Continued*)

Additive	Chemical	Form	Elemental	RDA	Dosage	Cost ($)
MINERALS—*continued*						
Magnesium sulfate	$MgSO_4$	IV, IM 1,000 mg/2 ml (50%)	48 (4 mEq) Mg/ml	280–350 mg	Mild magnesium deficiency: 1 g IM q 6 hr × 4 days Severe: 2.03/20 ml	0.79/2 ml
		10,000 mg/20 ml (10%)	9.6 mg (0.8 mEq) Mg/ml		2 mEq/kg IM or 5 g in 1 L D_5	
Magnesium oxide (Uro-Mag)		Capsule 140 mg	84.5 mg (7 m Eq) Mg/capsule	280–350 mg	3–4 capsules/day	0.46/capsule
Maalox Sodium-Free	Liquid 200 mg MgOH/5 ml	82 mg (6.8 mEq) Mg/5 ml	280–350 mg		0.79/180 ml	
Maalox Extra Strength Plus		Liquid 450 mg MgOH/5 ml	185 mg (15.4 mEq) Mg/5 ml	280–350 mg		1.08/5 oz
Maalox Plus		Tablet 200 mg MgOH	82 mg (6.8 mEq) Mg/tablet	280–350 mg	Chew 1–4 tablets, 4 times/day, 20–60 min after meals and at bedtime	0.17/tablet
Phosphorus						
Neutraphos		Sugar free fruit-flavored powder (75 ml reconstituted)	250 mg Phos 7.1 mEq Na/K	800–1200 mg	75 ml (2 1/2 oz) 4 times/day	0.29/packet

Sodium phosphate		IV 15 ml vial	93 mg Phos/ml 4 mEq Na/ml	800–1200 mg	1.91/15 ml
Potassium phosphate (K_2HPO_4)		IV 15 ml vial	93 mg Phos/ml 4.4 mEq K/ml	800–1200 mg	1.54/15 ml
Zinc					
Zinc chloride	$ZnCl_2$	IV 10 ml vial	1 mg Zn/ml	12–15 mg	Metabolically stable: 2.5–4.0 mg/day
					Catabolic: add 2 mg/day
					Small bowel output: 12.2 mg/L
Zinc sulfate		Capsule 220 mg	50 mg Zn/ capsule	12–15 mg	1 time/day	0.17 capsule

TABLE 13-2. Additional Additives

Additive	Chemical	Form	% of RDA	Ingredients	Dosage	Cost ($)
Multivitamins						
MVI-12		I.V.		100 mg vit C 1 mg vit A 5 μg vit D 3 mg vit B1 3.6 mg vit B2 4 mg vit B6 40 mg niacin 10 mg vit E 60 μg biotin 400 μg folic acid 5 μg vit B12 15 μg pantothenic acid (no vit K)	Vial 1 (5 ml) Vial 2 (5 ml)	
MTE-5		I.V.		1 mg zinc 0.4 mg copper 0.1 mg manganese 4 μg chromium 20 μg selenium	10 ml vial	2.53/10 ml

Therapeutic multivitamins with minerals	Tablet		0.12/tablet
	110% vit A	5,550 I.U.	
	200% vit C	120 mg	
	200% vit B1	3 mg	
	200% vit B2	3.4 mg	
	150% vit B6	3 mg	
	150% vit B12	9 µg	
	150% niacin	30 mg	
	100% vit D	400 I.U.	
	100% vit E	30 I.U.	
	100% pantothenic acid	10 mg	
	100% folic acid	0.4 mg	
	5% biotin	15 mcg	
	4% calcium	40 mg	
	100% iodine	150 µg	
	150% iron	27 mg	
	25% magnesium	100 mg	
	100% copper	2 mg	
	100% zinc	15 mg	
	100% manganese	5 mg	
	100% chromium	15 µg	
	100% Selenium	10 µg	
	100% Potassium	7.5 mg	
	100% Chloride	7.5 mg	

TABLE 13-2. (*Continued*)

Additive	Chemical	Form	% of RDA	Ingredients	Dosage	Cost ($)
Multivitamin Rowell		Soft gel	125% vit A 100% vit D 250% vit B1 208% vit B2 166% vit C 200% niacin Vit B6 Vit B12 Pantothenic acid Vit E	 0.5 mg 2 μg 5 mg 10 I.U.		0.08/tablet
Hexavitamin		Liquid	100% vit A 100% vit D 100% niacin 130% vit C 130% thiamin 180% riboflavin		5 ml	1.00/5 ml
Albee with C		Crushable tablet	500% vit C 1000% vit B1 600% vit B2 250% vit B6 250% niacin 100% pantothenic acid			0.12/tablet

B complex		Capsule	46% vit B1 41% vit B2 45% niacin 45% vit B6 33% vit B12	0.50/capsule
Sodium				
Sodium acetate	CH3COONa	16.4% 20 ml vial	2 mEq Na/ml 2 mEq HCO3/ml	5.52/20 ml
Sodium bicarbonate	NaHCO3	8.4% IV 50 ml vial	1 m Eq Na/ml 1 mEq HCO3/ml	1.78/50 ml
Sodium bicarbonate	NaHCO3	Tablet 650 mg	7.7 mEq Na/tablet 7.7 mEq HCO3/tablet	0.25/tablet
Sodium chloride	NaCl	0.9% IV 10 ml vial 20 ml vial	9 mg Mg/ml 9 mg Cl/ml	0.62/10 ml 1.54/20 ml
Sodium chloride	NaCl	Tablet 1 gm		0.17/tablet
Sodium chloride	NaCl	Table Salt	85.5 mEq Na/tsp 85.5 mEq Cl/tsp	
Sodium phosphate		IV	4 mEq Na/ml 93 mg Phos/ml	
Potassium				
Potassium acetate	CH3COOK	IV 19.6% 20 ml vial	2 mEq K/ml 2 mEq acetate/ml	1.58/20 ml

TABLE 13-2. (*Continued*)

Additive	Chemical	Form	% of RDA	Ingredients	Dosage	Cost ($)
Potassium bicarbonate (K-lyte)		Tablet 987 mg		25 mEq K/tablet		2.24/tablet
Potassium chloride	KCl	Oral solution 10% 15 ml		20 mEq K/15 ml		0.62/15 ml
Potassium chloride	KCl	IV 10 ml vial		2 mEq K/ml 2 mEq Cl/ml		0.87/10 ml
Potassium chloride	KCl	Tablet 10 mEq 20 mEq				0.40/tablet
Potassium phosphate		IV 15 ml vial		4.4 mEq K/ml 3 mmol P/ml		1.54/15 ml

Enteral Feeding Formulas and Administrative Techniques

CHAPTER

14

Patricia Heanue, R.D.

STEPS TAKEN PRIOR TO ADMINISTERING A TUBE FEEDING FORMULA

Prior to beginning formula administration, the following steps should be taken:

1. Verify all nasoenteric tube placements by x-ray. Those placed during a laparatomy need not be confirmed unless dislodgement is suspected.
2. Flush with 25 ml water to confirm patency.
3. Order enteral feeding pump and formula.
4. Begin feeding early in the hospital stay.
    Surgical patients
        Postpyloric tube—recovery room
        Intragastric tubes—24–48 h after surgery
    Medical: when appropriate

FORMULA ADMINISTRATION TECHNIQUES

Recently, we have conducted a prospective randomized, clinical trial of critically ill patients (serum albumin concentrations averaged 2.3 g/dl) receiving one of two enteral, elemental diets (1). No differences were noted between the amount of calories delivered and tolerance as assessed by diarrhea (more than three stools daily) and abdominal discomfort. The successful method used to administer diets in both groups was as follows.

1. Begin at 10 ml/hr and begin early in the course of therapy.
2. Use full-strength diets.
3. Increase gradually 10 ml/hr every 24 hr in the most critically ill and faster (e.g., 8 hr or 12 hr) in less severely ill patients. Do not remove venous access until fluid and metabolic needs can be met enterally. This is only a guideline. It is more important to start low volumes quickly than it is to advance quickly.
4. Monitor tolerance when formula administration begins. Refer to Chapter 16 for gastrointestinal complications and Chapter 15 for metabolic complications.
5. Check gastric residuals at least every 4 hr only if intragastric feeding is used. If the total volume of the residual exceeds 50% of the delivered formula *or* 150ml, reduce the rate of the formula in half. Do not check for residuals in the postpylorically fed patient.
6. Fiber (psyllium) is an excellent stool blinder and antidiarrheal agent but given its gelatinous nature should be taken orally (preferred) or bolused into a large-bore (>12 Fr) intragastric tube only. One packet of psyllium may be added to 4 (120 ml) to 8 oz (240 ml) of water.

Depending upon the patient's diagnosis and severity of illness, the routes of formula administration may be used as in Table 14-1.

SAMPLE OF ENTERAL FORMULA

A list of available formulas is presented in Table 14-2. Selected terms are defined here.

Polymeric formulas contain carbohydrate, protein, and fat in their natural form (high molecular weights). These require normal digestive and absorptive ability.

Elemental or predigested formulas contain at least one partially or totally digested macronutrient. Typically, elemental refers to the state of digestion of the protein source. This elemental or predigested formula may contain free amino acids and/or peptides, rather than intact protein molecules. Carbohydrate may be present as glucose and glucose polymers rather than as starch or maltodextrins. Formulas typically contain small amounts (<10 g/L) of long-chain triglycerides, but may contain up to 35% of the calories as a combination of medium-chain triglycerides (MCTs) and long-chain triglycerides (LCTs). These formulas may be beneficial to patients with compromised gastrointestinal (GI) tracts.

Enteral Feeding Formulas and Administrative Techniques 175

TABLE 14-1. Methods of Formula Delivery

	Pump		Bolus (Syringe or Gravity Drip)
Continuous	Discontinuous (Night Cycles, 8–12 hr)		
Usual Final Rates: 50–60 cc/hr	100–120 ml/hr		250 ml/bolus (1 can). Check residuals before initiating formula (should be < 50 ml)
Tube Tip Site Intragastric or postpyloric	Intragastric or postpyloric		Intragastric only
Patient Type Critically ill, comatosed, without gag reflex, risk of aspiration, bowel dysfunction	Stable patient		Alert, stable, usually ambulatory, intact GI tract
Oral Intake Unlikely due to sicker patient and continuously elevated insulin levels, which may curb appetite	Allows for increased activity during the day and reduced insulin levels, which may stimulate appetite		If oral diet is possible, adjust bolus meals so patient is able to consume orally as much as he or she wants.

Molecular components (e.g., protein, fat, carbohydrate, micronutrients) or "modular diets" are used to modify pre-existing commercial formulas with fixed macro- and micronutrient components. Addition of the modular component alters these fixed ratios.

Figure 14-1 shows a decision tree for formula selection.

SAMPLE TUBE FEEDING ORDERS

All tube feeding orders should include the following information: name of formula, strength, rate of administration, duration of time to administer.

Continuous Pump

Case: 78-year-old man male, s/p CABG could not be weaned from ventilator. Three weeks after coronary artery bypass graft, he underwent tracheostomy and the placement of a feeding jejunostomy tube.

TABLE 14-2. Sample of Enteral Formulas[a]

	Calories/ml	Protein (g/L)	Fat (g/L)	Carbohydrate (g/L)	Osmolality (mOsm/kg) H₂O	Sodium (mEq/L)	Potassium (mEq/L)	Volume to meet 100% RDA (ml)	Clinical indications	Comments	Flavors
Osmolite[b]	1.06	37 (14%)	38.5 (31%)	145 (55%)	300	23	26	1887	No severe organ dysfunction	Standard Tube Feeding (TF)	Unflavored
Sustacal[c]	1.01	61 (24%)	23 (21%)	140 (55%)	650	40	54	1060	Severely catabolic; suboptimal	TF or oral supplement, high-protein, high-potassium	Vanilla, chocolate
Sustacal[c] with Fiber	1.06	46 (17%)	35 (30%)	140 (53%)	480	31	36	1390	Long-term TF, Home TF	Fiber-containing TF or oral supplement (5.8 g fiber/L)	Chocolate, vanilla, strawberry
Vital HN[b]	1.0	41.7 (17%)	10.7 (9%)	185 (74%)	460	20.3	34.2	1500	GI dysfunction; transition to standard formula	Elemental low-fat TF, or oral supplement	Flavor packets available
Vivonex TEN[d]	1.0	38.2 (15%)	2.8 (3%)	206 (82%)	630	20	20	2000	GI dysfunction: transition to standard formula	Elemental low fat; low-potassium; contains free glutamine	Flavor packets available
Compleat[e]	1.07	43 (16%)	37 (31%)	141 (53%)	300	43	35.8	1500	No severe organ dysfunction	Standard TF Blenderized real food. Fiber containing	Unflavored
Impact[e]	1.0	56 (22%)	28 (25%)	132 (53%)	375	47	33	1500	Septic; severely, catabolic	Enriched with arginine & e fish oil; nucleotide containing	Unflavored

Product											
Magnacal[f]	2.0	70 (14%)	80 (36%)	250 (50%)	590	44	32	1000	Fluid restricted, patients i.e., renal failure, CHF	Low potassium	Vanilla
Hepatic[g] Aid II	1.2	44.1 (15%)	36.2 (28%)	169 (57%)	560	15	—	—	Patients w/ nitrogen or electrolyte retention disorders	TF or oral supplement	Chocolate
Ensure[b]	1.06	37 (14%)	37.2 (31.5%)	145 (54.5%)	470	36.8	40	1887	Suboptimal oral intake	Oral supplement	Vanilla, chocolate, strawberry, coffee
Ensure[b]	1.5	62 (17%)	50 (30%)	200 (53%)	650	51.3	46.6	947	Suboptimal oral intake catabolic patients	High-calorie high-protein oral supplement or tube feeding	Vanilla, chocolate
Carnation[h] Instant Breakfast (Whole Milk)	1.06	57 (22%)	31 (27%)	133 (51%)	700	45	60	1060	Suboptimal oral intake	Lactose-containing, high-protein oral supplement; available with whole, skim, or low-fat milk	Vanilla, chocolate, strawberry, coffee
Low-Sugar[h] Carnation Instant Breakfast (Whole Milk)	0.88	60 (28.%)	33.2 (34%)	81.6 (38%)	566	41	75	1000	Suboptimal oral intake; patients w/ DM	Contains Nutrasweet; lactose; high-protein; available with whole, skim, or low-fat milk; oral supplement	Vanilla, chocolate, coffee
Citrotein[e]	0.66	41 (25%)	1.6 (2%)	121 (73%)	480	31	18.2	1100	Suboptimal oral intake, patients requiring clear liquid diet	Clear liquid oral supplement	Punch, orange

TABLE 14-2. (Continued)

	Calories/ml	Protein (g/L)	Fat (g/L)	Carbohydrate (g/L)	Osmolality (mOsm/kg H$_2$O)	Sodium (mEq/L)	Potassium (mEq/L)	Volume to meet 100% RDA (ml)	Clinical indications	Comments	Flavors
Propac[f]	4/g	75%	8%	6%	—	9.8/100g	12.8/100g	—	Severely catabolic	Intact protein additive	Unflavored
MCT Oil[e]	7.7 (8.3/g)	—	100%	—	—	—	—	—	Not metabolized through intestinal lymphatics	Fat additive	Unflavored
Polycose[b] Powder	3.8/g	—	—	100%	—	—	—	—	Glucose polymer	Carbohydrate additive	Unflavored

[a] All products are lactose-free unless otherwise indicated.
[b] Ross Laboratories (Columbus, OH)
[c] Mead Johnson (Evansville, IN)
[d] Norwich Eaton Pharmaceuticals (Norwich, NY)
[e] Sandoz Nutrition (Minneapolis, MN)
[f] Sherwood Medical
[g] McGaw (Irvine, CA)
[h] Clintec Nutrition (Deerfield, IL)

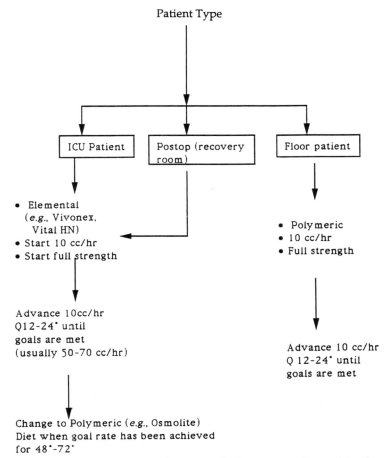

Figure 14-1. Decision tree for formula, rate, and advancement of enteral feeding.

Order: Day 1.

1. Full strength IMPACT (Sandoz, Minneapolis, MN) by feeding pump.
2.

Day	Rate of formula	Rate of IV
0-Recovery Room	10 ml/hr	TPN ($A_5D_{15}L_2$) 40 ml/hr
1	20 ml/hr	30 ml/hr
2	30 ml/hr	20 ml/hr
3	40 ml/hr	10 ml/hr
4	50 ml/hr	Discontinue IV

Discontinuous Pump

A 58-year-old woman with a history of Crohn's disease was admitted for numerous small bowel resections; feet of small bowel were remaining. Feeding jejunostomy was placed and patient was tolerating Sustacal, 60 ml/hr. Patient was ready to begin oral diet.

Order: Days 1 and 2. Diluted clear liquid diet. Full strength Sustacal (Mead Johnson, Evansville, IN) at:

Day	Rate of formula	Duration
1	80 ml/hr	18 hr (18:00–12:00)
2	120 ml/hr	12 hr (18:00–6:00)

Order: Day 3. Advance to full liquid (lactose-free, low-fat) diet. Full-strength Sustacal, 120 ml/hr (20:00–6:00).

Order: Day 4. Soft solids, low-fat, low-fiber, low-lactose; calorie counts. Full-strength Sustacal 80 ml/hr (20:00–6:00).

Order: Day 10. Discharge diet: soft solid, low-fat, low-fiber, low-lactose diet.

Oral caloric consumption < 1000 kcal/50 g protein. Full-strength Sustacal 100 ml/hr (20:00–6:00).

Bolus

A 78-year-old man had undergone total laryngectomy and was showing poor oral intake. He was admitted for rehydration and placement of a percutaneous endoscopic gastrostomy (PEG).

Order: Day 1.

1. 24-hours after PEG insertion, 20 ml bolus of D5W.
2. Full strength Osmolite 10 ml/hr for 6 hr. Increase by 10 ml/hr every 6 hr until goal of 60 ml/hr is achieved.
3. Bolus 300 ml at 7:00, 10:00, 13:00, 16:00, 19:00. Use this at home and increase amount of formula per feeding up to a maximum of 500 ml and reduce frequency to no fewer than 4 times per day.

REFERENCES

1. Borlase BC, Bell SJ, Lewis EJ, Swails W, Bistrian BR, Forse RA, Blackburn GL: Tolerance to enteral tube feeding diets in hypoalbuminemic, critically ill, geriatric patients: a prospective randomized trial. Surg Gynecol Obstet 1992, 174:181–188.

Metabolic Complications

CHAPTER 15

Kelli Guenther, R.D., CNSD

METABOLIC MONITORING AND TREATMENT

Appropriate monitoring of patients receiving enteral nutrition may decrease complications and facilitate successful provision of nutrition via feeding tubes. A suggested monitoring schedule is presented to ensure adequate, cost-effective monitoring (Table 15-1). Management of abnormalities is presented in Table 15-2.

REFEEDING SYNDROME

Several metabolic abnormalities, collectively termed the *refeeding syndrome*, may result during nutrient repletion of the marasmic or severely malnourished stressed patient. The syndrome is characterized by a shift of fluid and electrolytes as a result of insulin stimulation. Since marasmic patients have low levels of circulating insulin in the starved state, sudden elevation of insulin during the refeeding phase can result in antinaturesis and antidiuretic effects, causing expansion of extracellular fluid. Insulin also stimulates the intracellular uptake of phosphorus, potassium, and magnesium for lean tissue anabolism, causing depleted serum stores (reflected by low serum values), and often necessitating supplementation of $PO_4^=$, Mg^{++}, and K^+. Monitoring of patients most at risk for refeeding syndrome should focus on in/outs, daily weights, electrolytes (specifically $PO_4^=$, Mg^{++}, K^+, and blood glucose. Increases in fluid and calories should be gradual.

BIBLIOGRAPHY

APOVIAN CM, MCMAHON MM, BISTRIAN BR: Guidelines for refeeding the marasmic patient. Crit Care Med 18:1030–1033, 1990.

BRAUNWALD E, ISSELBACHER KJ, PETERSDORF RG, WILSON JD, MARTIN JB, FAUCI AS: Harrison's Principles of Internal Medicine. 11th ed. Companion Handbook. New York: McGraw-Hill, 1988, pp. 80–88.

KREY S, PORCELLI, K, LOCKETT G, KARLBERG P, SHRONTS E: Enteral nutrition, in Shronts EP (ed) Nutrition Support Dietetics: Core Curriculum. Rockville, MD: Aspen Publishers, 1989, pp. 63–81.

LENSSEN, PM: Monitoring and complications of parentereal nutrition, in Skipper A (ed) Dietitian's Handbook of Enteral and Parenteral Nutrition. Rockville, MD: Aspen Publishers, 1989, pp. 347–373.

SKIPPER A: Monitoring and complications of enteral feeding, in Skipper A (ed) Dietitian's Handbook of Enteral and Parenteral Nutrition. Rockville, MD: Aspen Publishers, 1989, pp. 293–309.

SOLOMON SM, KIRBY DF: The refeeding syndrome: a review. JPEN 14:90–97, 1990.

TABLE 15-1. Suggested Monitoring Schedule During Enteral Nutrition

Parameter		Frequency	Daily Cost ($)[a]
Serum albumin concentration	Baseline	q3 weeks	5.52
Weight	Baseline	PRN, at least weekly	—
In/Out		Daily	—
Na^+, K^+, Cl^-, CO_2, BUN, Creatinine	Baseline	PRN, at least weekly	43.86
Mg^{++}, Ca^{++}, PO_4	Baseline	Weekly	43.83
Blood glucose		PRN	6.90
Liver function tests (AST, ALT, LDH, alkaline phosphatase)	Baseline	PRN	44.16
24 hr urinary urea nitrogen		q 1–2 weeks	6.90
24 hr urine creatinine		q 1–2 weeks	8.97
Urine electrolytes		PRN	24.84
Total cost per week (if each test is done)			$185.00

[a] Costs are reflective of 1991 prices.

TABLE 15-2. Correction of Metabolic Complications During Enteral Nutrition Support[a]

Complication	Possible Cause	Management		
		Fluid	Tube Feeding	Medication
Hyperglycemia (maintain <200 mg/dl)	Diabetes Infection Corticosteroid therapy			Increase insulin dosage and/or use sliding scale
Hyponatremia (serum sodium <135 mEq/L)	Dilutional (congestive heart failure, edema, cirrhosis) Excess losses (gastrointestinal, renal)	Restrict free H_2O Replace losses parenterally Normal saline Lactated Ringer's	Use concentrated formula (e.g., Magnacal, (2 kCal/ml) Replace losses in tube feeding (TF) gradually. DO NOT BOLUS Add NaCl (85.5 mEq Na^+, 85.5 mEq Cl/teaspoon)	Diuretics (Sherwood Medical)
Hypernatremia (serum sodium >145 mEq/L)	Dehydration due to increased sensible/insensible fluid losses	Increase free H_2O		
Hypokalemia (serum potassium <3.5 mEq/L)	Metabolic alkalosis Excess losses, diuresis High-dosage insulin therapy Refeeding syndrome Amphotericin B, corticosteroid treatment	Replace losses parenterally KCl	Replace losses in TF gradually DO NOT BOLUS KCl (20 mEq K^+/15 ml) K-lite ($KHCO_3$) (25 mEq K^+, 25 mEq HCO_3/tablet)	

Condition	Causes		
Hypocalcemia (serum calcium <9.0 mg/dl)	Excess losses Vitamin D, Mg^{++}, parathyroid hormone PTH deficiency Hypoalbuminemia Aggressive PO_4 replacement Blood product transfusions		Supplement enterally based on ionized calcium –$CaCO_3$ (500 mg Ca^{++}/1250 mg tablet)
Hypercalcemia (serum calcium >11.0 mg/dl)	Aggressive antacid or vitamin D therapy Bone metastases Hyperparathyroidism	IV hydration	Diuresis
Hypomagnesium (serum magnesium <1.3 mEq/L)	Refeeding syndrome Excess losses Cisplatin, cyclosporine therapy	Replace losses parenterally: $MgSO_4$	Replace losses enterally Maalox (83 mg Mg^{++}/5ml) MgO (84 mg Mg^{++} capsule) $MgSO_4$ (192 mg Mg^{++}/1 g)
Hypermagnesemia (serum magnesium >3.0 mEq/L)	Renal insufficiency		Use low-magnesium formula Ensure (211 mg/1000 kCal) Osmolite (211 mg/1000 kCal) Magnacal (200 mg/1000 kCal) Vivonex TEN (200 mg/1000 kCal)

TABLE 15-2. (Continued)

Complication	Possible Cause	Management		
		Fluid	Tube Feeding	Medication
Hypocalcemia (serum calcium <9.0 mg/dl)	Excess losses Vitamin D, Mg^{++}, parathyroid hormone PTH deficiency Hypoalbuminemia Aggressive PO_4 replacement Blood product transfusions		Supplement enterally based on ionized calcium —$CaCO_3$ (500 mg Ca^{++}/1250 mg tablet)	
Hypercalcemia (serum calcium >11.0 mg/dl)	Aggressive antacid or vitamin D therapy Bone metastases Hyperparathyroidism	IV hydration		Diuresis
Hypomagnesium (serum magnesium <1.3 mEq/L)	Refeeding syndrome Excess losses Cisplatin, cyclosporine therapy	Replace losses parenterally: $MgSO_4$	Replace losses enterally Maalox (83 mg Mg^{++}/5ml) MgO (84 mg Mg^{++} capsule) $MgSO_4$ (192 mg Mg^{++}/1 g)	
Hypermagnesemia (serum magnesium >3.0 mEq/L)	Renal insufficiency		Use low-magnesium formula Ensure (211 mg/1000 kCal) Osmolite (211 mg/1000 kCal) Magnacal (200 mg/1000 kCal) Vivonex TEN (200 mg/1000 kCal)	

Condition	Cause		Treatment
Low serum zinc (serum zinc <55 mg/dl)	Excess losses	Replace losses parenterally	Replace losses enterally: ZnSO$_4$ (50 mg Zn^{++}/capsule)
Azotemia	Dehydration	Increase free H$_2$O	Maintain adequate protein intake (1.5 g/kg IBW)
	Catabolism		
	Renal insufficiency		Dialysis
Metabolic acidosis	Renal failure		Replace losses in TF gradually, DO NOT BOLUS NaHCO$_3$ (7.7 mEq Na$^+$, 7.7 mEq HCO$_3$/tablet)
	Drug therapy (amphotericin-B, aminoglycosides)		
	Excess HCO$_3$ losses		
	Diabetic/starvation ketoacidosis		Increase insulin
Metabolic alkalosis	Excess Cl$^-$ losses	Replace losses parenterally	Replace losses in TF gradually, DO NOT BOLUS NaCl CaCl KCl
	Corticosteroid therapy		
	Blood product transfusion		

[a]Refer to Chapter 3 for further dosage recommendations for nutritional replacement.

CHAPTER 16

Gastrointestinal Complications: Diarrhea and High Gastric Residuals

Shanthi Thomas, M.S., R.D., CNSD

DIARRHEA

Gastrointestinal complications can be minimized by the appropriate selection of access routes into the gastrointestinal (GI) tract. For the most satisfactory results, we suggest feeding past the pylorus or, more specifically, past the ligament of Trietz. This virtually eliminates gastric discomfort, nausea and vomiting, and pulmonary aspiration.

Diarrhea may be defined as >500 ml stool output over a 24 hr period or more than 3 stools/day. The type (polmeric vs. elemental) of tube feeding formula is rarely the cause. Moreover, it is unnecessary to stop the tube feeding formula until the cause is identified.

The following major causes of diarrhea are listed in descending order of frequency. Many elixirs contain sorbitol, frequently in laxative dosages that cause diarrhea by stimulating GI motility and increasing the secretory process. If possible, consider use of a nonelixir form, or give medication intravenously.

High Osmotic Load. A high osmotic load (>1000 mOs/kg) may occur from additives to the tube-feeding formula.

Other medications that may markedly increase osmolality and/or irritate the GI tract include magnesium antacids, cimetidine, potassium and phosphorus supplements, quinidine compounds, lactulose, and various laxatives. (Every mEq is equivalent to 1 mOsm/kg. Thus, 50 mEq KCl is an extra 100 mOsm/kg to the final osmolality of the tube feeding formula (50 for the K^+, 50 for the Cl^-).

If medications are suspected as the contributing factor (either sorbitol content or high osmolality)

1. Change to nonelixir form/review medication for need
2. If possible, do not bolus medication but mix with tube feeding diet throughout day and administer every 4–6 hr
3. For known GI irritants such as quinidine and magnesium compounds, change to parenteral administration when applicable, or use a nonirritating, alternative medication.

Antibiotic Administration. Diarrhea may be common in enterally fed patients receiving antibiotics, primarily due to altered colonization of the GI tract.

Treatment of Diarrhea

Proper treatment of diarrhea is dependent on the cause. If *Clostridium difficile* is suspected as the offending pathogen, obtain *Clostidium difficile* toxin assay. In addition, test stool cultures for ova and parasites. If stool culture is positive for *C. difficile* start vancomycin at a dosage of 125–250 mg four times daily for 10–14 days. The IV dosage of vancomycin may vary, depending upon the patient's renal function. If stool culture is negative for *C. difficile,* the patient may be started on Lomotil or deoderized tinture of opium. Refer to Table 16-1 for dosage and administration guidelines. If diarrhea continues to be severe, patients may benefit from parenteral (peripheral or central) alimentation.

HIGH GASTRIC RESIDUALS

Causes

Causes are only a problem if the patient is fed intragastrically. Do not attempt to aspirate back and measure residuals in patients fed postpylorically. Because of the risk of aspiration feeding, intragastric is not recommended for patients in the intensive care unit (ICU). Major causes of delayed gastric emptying are sepsis, elevated blood sugar levels, diabetic gastroparesis, diabetic gastroparesis, elevated body temperature, ischemia or surgical repairs, and the formula fat content. Many drugs have been implicated in reducing the gastric emptying (Table 16-2). Osmolality of the tube feeding formula is unlikely to be the major

TABLE 16-1. Guidelines for Lomotil/Deoderized Tinture of Opium: Use in Enteral Formulas

Stool Volume (ml)	Lomotil Dosage[a] (ml/L formula)	D.T.O. Dosage[a,b] (gtts/L formula)	Psyllium[c] (Fiber); bolus directly per NG tube only (packets)
100–250 (nondiarrhea)	10	5	1
250–500 (nondiarrhea)	15	10	1–2
500–1000 (diarrhea)	20	15	2–3
>1000 (diarrhea)		Reduce or terminate enteral infusion	

[a]Add Lomotil or DTO directly to formula; do not bolus separately.
[b]20 qtts = 1.0 ml.
[c]Do not add directly to the tube feeding formula, since it forms a gel and may clog the tube. A large-bore (>12 Fr) gastric tube (nasogastric or gastrostomy) is required for successful administration. Best results are obtained by mixing with water (4–8 oz) and bolusing directly into the tube. It is important to flush with water (>50–100m) after administration. Only intragastrically fed patients may receive psyllium due to the large amount of water that needs to be bolused during administration.

For patients receiving a low-carbohydrate diet (e.g., diabetics), sugar-free psylium may be used. Also, a fiber-enriched enteral formula may be tried (refer to Chapter 14).

cause. If high residuals appear or delayed emptying is suspected, add a few drops of methylene blue to the tube feeding formula daily to trace the route of formula (e.g., into lungs) until the problem resolves. Aspiration is rare in patients fed postpylorically and this method of feeding is advocated for all critically ill patients.

Treatment

The following protocol is used for the treatment of gastric residuals.

1. Check gastric residuals every 4 hr.
2. If residuals are greater than two times the tube feeding rate, decrease the rate.
3. Begin with IV Reglan, followed by enteral route (oral or added to formula). If IV access is unavailable, use the oral, liquid form added to the formula. The most commonly prescribed dosage for Reglan is 10 mg four times daily (oral/IV).
4. The formula is unlikely to be a contributing factor unless any of the following are present: osmolality (> 650 mOs/kg), fat (long-chain triglycerides) content (> 10% total calories), or, rate (patient receiving more than 25–30 kCal/kg).

TABLE 16-2. Factors that Influence Gastric Emptying (GE)

Pathologic Factors	Increase GE	Decrease GE
Acute abdomen		+
Chronic calculous	+	
Laparotomy		+
Trauma and pain		+
Labor		+
Myocardial infarction		+
Gastric ulcer		+
Duodenal ulcer	+	
Hepatic coma		+
Hypercalcemia		+
Diabetes mellitus		+
Myxedema		+
Malnutrition		+
Migraine		+
Raised intracranial pressure		+
Atrophic gastritis: solids		+
Astrophic gastritis: liquids	+	
Pyloric stenosis		+
Gastric volvulus		+
Intestinal obstruction		+
Gastroenterostomy	+	
Anticholinergic drugs		
Atropine		+
Propantheline		+
Tricyclics		+
Trihexyphenidyl		+
Ganglion-blocking drugs:		
Hexamethonium		+
Narcotic analgesics		
Morphine		+
Pentazocine		+
Isoniazid		+
Sodium nitrate		+
Chloroquine		+
Alcohol		+
Dioctyl sodium sulfosuccinate		+
Phenytoin		+
Metoclopramide	+	
Reserpine	+	
Anticholinesterases	+	
Sodium bicarbonate	+	

continued on next page

TABLE 16-2. *(Continued)*

Pathologic Factors	Increase GE	Decrease GE
Aluminum hydroxide		+
Magnesium hydroxide		+
Liquids	+	
Solids		+
Acid		+
Fat		+
Increased osmotic pressure		+
Amino acids		+
Gastric distention	+	
Gastrin		+
Secretin		+
Cholecystokinin		+
Glucagon		+
Posture (prone or right side)	+	

Adapted from Nimmo WS: Clin Pharmacokinet 1:189–203, 1976.

If increased gastric residuals persist, the patient may benefit from postpyloric feedings. The gastroenterology service may put in a percutaneous endoscopic gastrostomy–jejunostomy or a surgeon may create a surgical jejunostomy.

BIBLIOGRAPHY

Edes-Thomas E, Walk-Betty E, Austin JL: Diarrhea in tube-fed patients: feeding formula not necessarily the cause. JAMA 88:91–93, 1990.

Haynes-Johnson V: Tube feeding complications: causes, prevention, and therapy. Nutr Supp Serv 6:17–24, 1986.

Heimburger-Douglas C: Diarrhea with enteral feeding: Will the real cause please stand up? JAMA 89–90, 1990.

Krey H, Murray RL: Dynamics of Nutrition Support, Assessment, Implementation, Evaluation. Norwalk, CT: Appleton-Century-Crofts, 1986.

Lang CE: Nutritional Support in Critical Care. Rockville, MD: ASPEN, 1987.

Rombeau JL, Caldwell MD: Clinical Nutrition Enteral and Tube Feeding, 2nd edition. Philadelphia: W.B. Saunders, 1990.

Feeding Tube Placement

CHAPTER 17

*Bradley C. Borlase, M.D., M.S.
and R. Armour Forse, M.D., Ph.D.*

SURGICAL TUBE PLACEMENT

Selection of the correct site of placement for the feeding tube is an important aspect of ensuring success with enteral nutrition. Patients in the intensive care unit (ICU), without exception, are best fed postpylorically. The first choice in geriatric, critically ill patients is to place the tube surgically by the methods shown in Figure 17-1. There were no major complications using this technique. However, this procedure is mostly reserved for patients undergoing a laparatomy for their primary disease and for whom there is no increased risk of an enterostomy. Otherwise, patients may receive a gastrostomy with a postpyloric tube threaded through it. In less critically ill patients and those requiring long-term tube feedings (e.g., patients with head and neck cancer), a gastrostomy tube may be placed.

TRANSNASAL TUBE PLACEMENT

The next best choice is to pass an 8 Fr, 43 inch long feeding tube transnasally during surgery. This procedure would be suitable for surgical patients who are

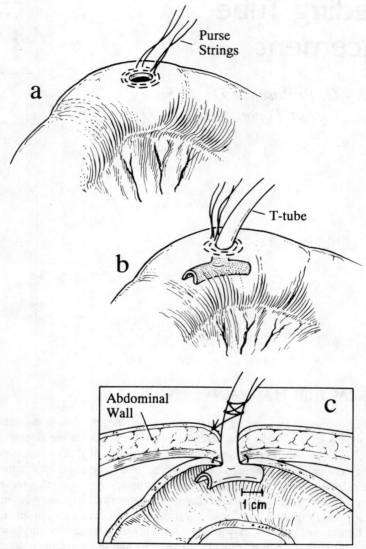

Figure 17-1. *Step A* Isolate segment of the jejunum 2 feet from the Ligament of Trietz which rests comfortably to the abdominal wall. Place 2 purse string sutures in the antimesenteric boarder of the jejunum. Make a controlled, enterotomy within the purse string sutures. Fashion the biliary tube as a standard T-tube.

Step B Cut the tips so that each side is 1 cm in length. Place the tube (tip end) into the jejunum and tie the purse strings.

Step C Use 4 tacking sutures to the abdominal wall. Patient may be fed in the recovery room.

immunocompromised (due to acquired immunodeficiency syndrome [AIDS], transplantation, inflammatory bowel disease) have a coagulopathy, or violation of the gastrointestinal (GI) tract is of concern to the surgeon. The tip of the tube (e.g., Keofeed) should pass the ligament of Trietz. Nasojejunal tubes, as with all other tubes, can inadvertently become dislodged and it may be appropriate to secure the tube to the nose.

Transnasal intubation may be performed at bedside using IV metaclopamide (Reglan) administered to stimulate peristalsis. Endoscopic placement is a viable alternative if one encounters difficulty in passing the tube through the pylorus.

Intragastric access is most readily achieved transnasally with an 8 Fr, 36 inch long feeding tube, but should be used to feed noncritically ill patients for whom the risk of aspiration is minimal.

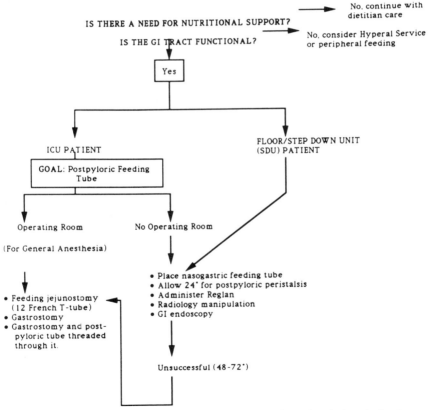

Figure 17-2. Decision trees for selection of enteral feeding tubes in hospitalized patients.

PERCUTANEOUS TUBE PLACEMENT

A percutaneous endoscopic gastrostomy (PEG) may be placed safely. A small feeding tube may be threaded through the PEG by use of an endoscope to allow for postpyloric feedings. Patients can be fed distally with simultaneous gastric suction. For critically ill patients not requiring a laparotomy, a PEG–jejunostomy is an excellent method for successful enteral feeding. Once the patient is stabilized and leaves the unit, the jejunostomy portion may be removed, and the patient fed intragastrically.

DECISION TREE FOR TUBE PLACEMENT

Figure 17-2 shows the decision tree used by our enteral service in selecting feeding tubes and placement sites.

REFERENCES

1. Borlase BC, Babineau, TJ, Forse RA, Bell SJ, Blckburn GL: Enteral nutrition support, in Rippe JM, Irwin RS, Alpert JS, Fink MP (eds.), Intensive Care Medicine. Boston: Little, Brown, 1991, pp. 1669–1674.

Care of Feeding Tubes

CHAPTER 18

Ann Thibault, R.N., CNSN

CARE OF SURGICAL TUBE SITE

Clean the site daily with half-strength hydrogen peroxide or full-strength providone–iodine. Check the site for redness, drainage, and proper anchorage of tube. Apply the dry sterile dressing (DSD) daily. Routine care of the feeding tube may be done by the patient's nurse without a physician's order.

HOW TO UNCLOG A FEEDING TUBE

Try to avoid the problem: Always flush the tube with 20ml warm water when feeding is stopped, interrupted, before and after medication. You cannot overdo this procedure

If true clogging occurs: order 'papain 2.5% solution as directed' from the pharmacy. Papain, an enzyme derived from pineapple, hydrolyzes protein (a major component of enteral diets and the most likely cause of clogging). An improperly crushed pill may cause the clogging, in which case papain will have no effect.

When using papain 2.5%, follow these steps:

1. Using a syringe, instill 1–5ml of the papain solution into the feeding tube, or as much of the 5ml as you can get in.
2. Let the solution sit in the feeding tube for 30 min.
3. After 30 min, attempt to flush the tube with warm water. Repeat steps 1 and 2 up to three times.

If these steps fail, order a guidewire (0.035 mm). A physician may gently insert the wire to clear obstruction. Check patency using x-ray examination.

MEDICATION ADMINISTRATION

Medications should always be given by vein or orally, unless it is absolutely necessary to give medication via the feeding tube.

When providing medications via the feeding tube, follow these steps:

1. Only electrolytes, vitamins, and minerals should be added directly to the tube feeding formula (e.g., NaCl, KCl, $NaOH_3$, $CaCl_2$, multivitamin, etc.).
2. Bolus administer other medications (finely crushed and mixed with 20ml warm water). The tube feeding must be stopped during administration of medications. Flush the tube with 20ml warm water before and after administration of medication.
3. Most medications (nonelectrolytes) are absorbed in the duodenum, so avoid administering them via a jejunostomy.
4. Do not give enteric-coated or sustained-released medications via any feeding tube.
5. Syrups high in alcohol often result in coagulation of the enteral formula, causing a clogged tube.

Transitional Feeding Strategies for Discharge

CHAPTER 19

Elaine B. Trujillo, M.S., R.D., CNSD

DEFINITION OF TERMS

Transitional feeding is the act of advancing from one route of feeding to another or from one formula to another. The key factor in making a successful transition includes the provision of optimal nutrients during the transitional period. In this chapter, we discuss the modalities of transitional feeding typically encountered, as shown in Figure 19-1.

TRANSITION FROM ONE TUBE FEEDING FORMULA TO ANOTHER

The guidelines for making transitions between tube feeding (TF) formulas are given in Table 19-1.

TRANSITION FROM TUBE FEEDING TO AN ORAL DIET

Patients with Impaired Gut Function or Who Have Not Taken an Oral Diet for Over 1 Month

Most patients, except those with severe strokes or mechanical problems which prevent oral ingestion of food, are able to consume an oral diet eventually. The longer a patient has been without an oral diet, the longer the transition phase (Table 19-2). We suggest a slow progress (approximately 3 weeks) for patients with impaired gut function but able to take an oral diet; prolonged time without oral intake (NPO) (> 1 month); gastrointestinal (GI) intolerance while receiving tube feeding diet; major gastrointestinal surgery.

Patients with a Normal Gastrointestinal Tract Who Have Consumed an Oral Diet Within 1 Month

Patients with normal gut function (and who usually have consumed an oral diet within 1 month) may begin on a full liquid diet when ready, rather than taking a traditional, clear liquid diet first. If this is tolerated over the first 24 hr, the diet should be advanced to solid food. Calorie counts should be initiated once the patient is taking a full liquid diet.

Cyclic Tube Feedings

Cycling the tube feedings, usually at night, improves the patient's appetite and often allows for increased ambulation. Cyclic tube feedings should begin when the patient begins eating solid food. The usual practice in initiating cyclic feedings is as shown in Table 19-3.

Discontinuation of Tube Feeds

Once the patient is consuming two-thirds to three-quarters of protein and energy needs orally, consistently over a 3-day period, and gives the impression that he or she can nourish and hydrate adequately, the tube feeding formula may be stopped. If a nasoenteric tube is present, it can be removed. If a permanent access tube is present, it should be capped and flushed regularly to preserve patency. It should not be removed until the patient's first return visit to the physician as an outpatient.

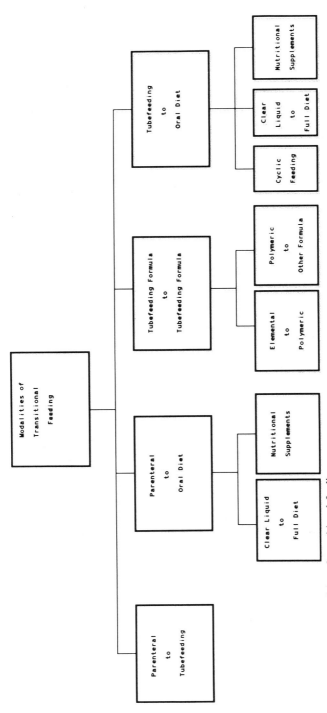

Figure 19-1. Modalities of transitional feeding.

TABLE 19-1. Guidelines for Transition Between Tube Feeding Formulas

Transition	Indications	Rationale	Guidelines[a]
Elemental to polymeric formula	Patient tolerating elemental TF formula without evidence of nausea, vomiting, abdominal discomfort, or diarrhea	Composition similar to real food Prepares the patient to eat Less cost Less preparation	Day 1: 3/4 elemental, 1/4 polymeric Day 2: 1/2 elemental, 1/2 polymeric Day 3: 1/4 elemental, 3/4 polymeric Day 4: Full-strength polymeric
Polymeric to fiber formula	Patient tolerating standard polymeric formula	Long-term care Constipation Diarrhea[b]	Day 1: 1/2 polymeric, 1/2 polymeric with fiber Day 2: Full-strength polymeric with fiber
Polymeric to other formulas	Patient tolerating current polymeric formula	Alternative nutrient composition desired (e.g., high-protein, low-fat, low-potassium) Alternative formula (e.g., more convenient, less cost, etc.)	Patients who have been stable can make the transition in one day, replacing one formula with another Patients who have experienced intolerance to TFs should make the transition in 2 days Day 1: 1/2 polymeric, 1/2 new formula Day 2: Full-strength new formula

[a] Usual practice is that admixtures, such as protein module (e.g., Propac [Sherwood Medical], vitamins, and minerals should be added once at full strength, because clumping has been known to occur. Other additives necessary for metabolic management (e.g., NaCl) should continue to be added during the transition process. The transition guidelines should be run at the desired TF rate.

[b] Diarrhea secondary to an infection or medication should be ruled out before initiating use of a fiber-supplemented TF formula.

TABLE 19-2. Progression from a Tube Feeding Diet to an Oral Diet in Patients with Impaired Gut Function

Day 1	1/2 strength clear liquid diet[a], maintain same rate of tube feeding formula
Day 2	(Or when indicated): full liquid diet[b] (lactose-free, low fat). Begin to taper tube feeding diet. Begin calorie counts.
Day 3	(Or when indicated): regular or therapeutic diet. Stop tube feeding when patient consumes two thirds to three fourths of protein and energy needs for 3 days.

[a]Clear liquids are indicated initially but should be diluted to half strength due to the hyperosmolar nature of these beverages. The osmolalities of some clear liquids are presented in Table 9-1, Chapter 9.

[b]A full liquid diet usually follows a clear liquid diet. However, some patients, particularly those who have not been exposed to lactose-containing products for over a month, are unable to tolerate full liquid diets. For these patients, use lactose-free supplements, or add the lactase to reduce lactose content of these products, and/or advance to a solid diet, with an increased variety of foods. A low-fat diet is indicated in patients with a known fat intolerance. Lactose-free milk and other milk products are available.

TABLE 19-3. Progression of 24-Hr/Day Tube Feeding to Reduced Schedule[a]

Day 1	Cycle over 18 hr (e.g., 18:00–12:00)
Day 2	Decrease cycle to 12 hr (e.g. 20:00–8:00)
Day 3	Decrease cycle to 8 or 10 hr or desired time period (e.g., 20:00–6:00)

[a]Increase the rate of formula to meet the desired caloric goal.

DAILY GASTROINTESTINAL TOLERANCE MONITORING DURING TRANSITION

Monitoring gastrointestinal tolerance during the transition should involve evaluation of the following:

1. Diarrhea, gastric residuals (patients with intragastric tube feedings only), abdominal distention, nausea, vomiting, swallowing, and signs of malabsorption.
2. Calorie counts
3. If the patient has a tracheostomy or has had a prolonged period of intubation, check for signs of dysphagia, aspiration, and discomfort on swallowing.

PREPARE PATIENT FOR DISCHARGE

For a patient to be discharged to chronic care or home, a permanent feeding access is required. Oral intake may progress while the patient is receiving tube

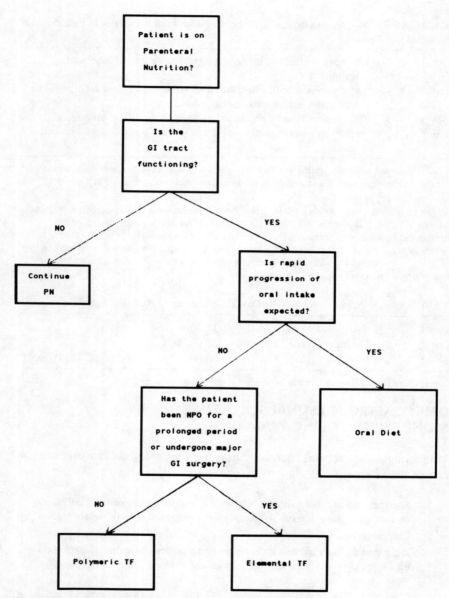

Figure 19-2. Transitioning from parenteral to enteral nutrition.

feeding diets. In many cases, this can shorten the length of hospital stay by not forcing the patient to meet nutritional needs orally before being discharged.

Strategies for Discharging a Patient Receiving a TF Diet

1. Change to appropriate formula, if indicated. Refer to Chapter 14 for formula selection.
2. Make transition to cyclic feeding. Refer to Table 19-3 for guidelines.
3. Contact a home health care agency if patient requires a feeding pump, formula, and/or nursing care. A consultation may usually be initiated by any member of the health care team.

Options for Permanent Feeding Tubes and Method of Administration

1. Gastrostomy tube: pump, bolus, or gravity drip
2. Jejunostomy tube: pump or gravity drip (in selected cases)

Guidelines for Discontinuing TF at home

1. Continue to use tube feeding diet until the patient consumes at least two-thirds to three-quarters of calorie and protein requirements, as assessed by a dietitian.
2. Use a team approach (nurse/physician/dietitian) to determine when to remove the feeding tube.

BIBLIOGRAPHY

BELL SJ, ANDERSON FL, BISTRIAN BR, DANNER EH, BLACKBURN GL: Osmolality of beverages commonly provided on clear and full liquid menu. Nutr Clin Pract 2:241–244, 1987.

KREY SH, MURRAY RL: Modular and transitional feedings, in Rombeau JL, Caldwell MD (eds) Enteral and Tube Feedings. Philadelphia: W.B. Saunders, 1990, pp. 127–148.

PARADIS KM, BELL SJ, BENOTTI PN: Transitional feeding in small bowel resection, in Blackburn GL, Bell SJ, Mullen JL (eds) Nutritional Medicine: A Case Management Approach. Philadelphia: W.B. Saunders, 1989, pp. 73–77.

WADE J: Parenteral and enteral transition techniques, in Krey SH, Murray RL (eds) Dynamics of Nutrition Support: Assessment, Implementation, Evaluation. East Norwalk, CT: Appleton & Lange, 1986, pp. 489–496.

ZIBRIDA JM, CARLSON S: Transitional feeding, in Shonts E (ed) Nutritional Support Core Curriculum. Silver Spring, MD: ASPEN Publishers, 1989, pp. 287–294.

Index

A

Abbott, W. O., 79
Abdominal Trauma Index (ATI), 84
Acalculous cholecystitis, 30
Acute care, advancement to chronic care from, 67, 203, 205
Alanine, 88
Albumin, 82
Alexander, J. W., 17, 49
Alexander, W., 88
Al-Saady, N. M., 124
Alverdy, J., 19
American Society for Parenteral and Enteral Nutrition (A.S.P.E.N.), 29, 63, 127, 155
Amin-Aid, 122, 123
Andrassy, Richard J., 15–21, 20
Andressen, A. F. R., 79
Antibiotics, 17–18, 20, 131, 189

Arginine, 19–20, 48–49
Askanazi, J., 122

B

Babineau, Timothy J., 47–54
Bacterial microflora, 17–18, 27–29
Bacterial translocation, 8, 15–21, 29, 31–33, 50, 87–91, 107–8
Barbul, A., 48, 49
Basal Energy Expenditure (BEE), 156–57
Bell, Stacey J., 63–67, 69–76, 142–50
Bessman, A. N., 120
Beverage osmolalities, 111, 112
Bistrian, Bruce R., 53, 73, 142–50
Blackburn, George L., 63–67, 73, 142–50
Blood, in stools, 131
Border, J. R., 85

Borlase, Bradley C., 63–67, 69–76, 142–50, 193–98
Bowel obstruction, 64
Branched-chain stress formulas, 127, 128
Breath hydrogen analysis, 31
Brush border enzymes, 28
Burke, D. J., 19
Burn formulas, 127, 128
Butyrate, 28

C

Calcium additives, 164–65
Caloric requirements, 39–40, 156–58
Carbohydrate requirements, 42–43, 158, 159
Carbohydrate-restricted formulas, 122, 124, 125
Cardiac stability, 32
Catabolic illness, formulas for, 127, 128
Catheters, 65–66
Cerra, F. B., 50–51, 127
Chiu, C. J., 6
Christie, M. L., 119
Chronic care, advancement from acute care to, 67, 203, 205
Concentrated formulas, 124, 126
Critical illness, 25–34
 bacterial translocation and, 29, 31–33, 50
 GI tract as source of stress, 26–27
 indications for enteral nutrition, 29–33
 stress effects on GI tract, 26–27
Crockett, Christine, 115–36
Cuthbertson, D. P., 5, 80
Cyclic feeding, 111, 200, 203

D

Daly, J. M., 48
Dascoulias, Kathy, 69–76
Deitch, E. A., 16–18
Delany, H. M., 79, 92
Dextrose, 43
Diabetes formulas, 124
Diamond, J. M., 6
Diarrhea, 30, 32, 43, 72, 75, 131, 134–36, 188–90
Digestion, 3–4

Dudrick, S. J., 69, 80
Duodenal secretions, 4

E

Edsal, D. L., 79
Egberts, E. H., 119–20
Electrolyte additives, 161, 171–72
Elemental (predigested) formulas, 65, 116, 118, 135, 136, 174, 202
Elman, R., 80
Endotoxins, 8–9, 17, 18, 29, 31, 33
Ensure Plus, 124, 126
Enteral feeding formulas, 115–36
 administration of, *see* Enteral feeding technique
 branched-chain stress, 127, 128
 carbohydrate-restricted, 122, 124, 125
 concentrated, 124, 126
 decision tree for selection, 117
 diarrhea and, 131, 134–36
 elemental (predigested), 65, 116, 118, 135, 136, 174, 202
 fiber-containing, 135, 136, 202
 hepatic, 116, 119–21
 immune-enhancing, 127, 128
 initial assessment, 115–16
 micronutrient additives, 161–72
 polymeric, 65, 174, 202
 protein, 127, 129, 130, 132–33
 renal, 120, 121, 123
 sample of, 174–78
 selection of, 65
 strength of, 66
 See also Nutritional requirements
Enteral feeding technique, 63–67, 173–74
 advancement from acute to chronic care, 67, 203, 205
 delivery methods, 175
 feeding tubes
  care of, 197–98
  placement of, 193–98
  selection of, 65–66
 formula selection, 65
 formula strength, 66
 gastrointestinal complications, 188–92
  diarrhea, 30, 32, 43, 72, 75, 131, 134–36, 188–90
  high gastric residuals, 189–92

infusion rate, 66–67
initiation of, 65
metabolic complications, 181–86
patient selection criteria, 64–65, 155–56
sample tube feeding orders, 175, 179–80
steps prior to administration, 173
transitional feeding, *see* Transitional feeding
See also Enteral feeding formulas
Enteral Nutrition Service (ENS), 69–76
daily activities, 71–72
formation of, 70–71
justification of, 72, 75–76
nutritional status assessment, 74–75
operational decision tree, 73
Enteral nutrition technique, *see* Enteral feeding technique
Enterocyte function, 4–9, 27–28

F

Farquhar, M. G., 6
Fats, *see* Lipids
Federation of American Societies for Experimental Biology, 127
Feeding tubes
care of, 197–98
placement of, 193–98
selection of, 65–66
Felli, Franaseo, 79
Fenton, J. C. B., 120
Fiber-containing formulas, 135, 136, 202
Fiber polysaccharides, intraluminal fermentation of, 28
Fisher, J. E., 116, 119
Fish oils, 43, 53, 54, 159
Folic acid additive, 165
Formulas, *see* Enteral feeding formulas
Forse, R. Armour, 63–67, 69–76, 142–50, 193–98
Fox, A. D., 51

G

Gastric emptying, 189–92
Gastric secretions, 4
Gastrointestinal complications, 188–92

diarrhea, 30, 32, 43, 72, 75, 131, 134–36, 188–90
high gastric residuals, 189–92
Gastrointestinal failure, 4
Gastrointestinal tolerance monitoring, 203
Gastrointestinal tract
bacterial translocation and, 8, 15–21, 29, 31–33, 50, 87–91, 107–8
critical illness and, 25–34
bacterial translocation, 29, 31–33, 50
GI tract as source of stress, 26–27
indications for enteral nutrition, 29–33
stress effects, 26–27
hypermetabolic response to injury and, 3–11, 50
enterocyte function, 4–9
systemic response, 8–10
See also Postoperative feeding
nutritional requirements and, *see* Nutritional requirements
Glucerna, 124, 125
Glucose, 42–43
Glutamine, 19, 28, 32, 49–51, 88
Gram-negative bacteria, 18, 20, 27
Guenther, Kelli, 181–186
Gumbiner, B., 6
Gut-associated lymphoid tissue (GALT), 28

H

Harris-Benedict equations, 39, 157
Harvey, William, 79
Hayashi, J. T., 149
Heanue, Patricia, 173–180
Hemorrhagic shock, bacterial translocation and, 16–17, 19
Henrique, V., 80
Hepatic Aid, 119–21
Hepatic-Aid II, 161, 177
Hepatic formulas, 116, 119–21
Heymsfield, S. B., 122
High gastric residuals, 189–92
High nitrogen formulas, 127, 129, 130
High osmotic load, 188–89
Hormonal factors in epithelial cell growth, 4
Horst, D., 119
Hypercatabolic illness, enteral products for, 127, 128
Hypercatabolism, 82

Hypermetabolic response to injury, 3–11, 50
  enterocyte function, 4–9
  systemic response, 8–10
  See also Postoperative feeding, early
Hyperosmolality, 135
Hypertonic formulas, 136
Hypoalbuminemic patients, 135
Hypomotility agents, 135–36
Hypothermia, 5
Hypovolemia, 5

I

Ileus, 26–27, 30, 32
ImmunAid, 127, 128
Immune defenses, impaired, 18–19
Immune-enhancing formulas, 127, 128
Impact, 127, 128, 176
Indirect calorimetry, 40, 84–85
Inflammatory response, 8
Infusion rate, 66–67
Injury, hypermetabolic response to, *see* Hypermetabolic response to injury
Insulin, 181–82
Interdigestive motor complex (IMC), loss of, 26–27
Interleukin-1, 66, 81, 87
Intestinal microflora, alteration of, 17–18, 28–29
Intestinal obstruction, 18
Iron additives, 165
Isoleucine, 41–42
Isotonic formulas, 136

J

Jaundice, obstructive, 18
Jejunostomy feeding, 65–66
  placement, 92–94
  postoperative management, 94–96
  study of associated complications, 142–50
Jensen, Gordon L., 3–11
Jones, B. J. M., 65
Jones, Todd N., 78–101

K

Kane, R. E., 124
Khoury, Thomas L., 142–50
King, Sir Edward, 79
Kinney, John M., 122
Kulkarni, A. D., 52

L

Lactose, digestion of, 135
Lebow, Martha, 155–59
Leucine, 41–42
Leukotrienes, 53
Linoleic acid, 53, 159
Lipids
  metabolism following injury, 81–82
  requirements for, 43, 159
  structured, 52–54
Liver disease, 116, 119–20
Lomotil, 189, 190
Long-chain triglycerides (LCTs), 43, 52–54, 174
Loran, M. R., 4
Lowen, Richard, 79

M

Ma, L., 17
MacDonald, A. H., 79
Macronutrient requirements, 40–43, 156–59
Madara, J. L., 6–7
Magnesium additives, 165–66
Maintenance feeding, long-term, 129
Maldigestion, 116
Mascioli, E. A., 54
McGhee, A., 119
Medication administration, 198
Medium-chain triglycerides (MCT), 43, 52–54, 159, 174
Metabolic assessment, 82–85
Metabolic complications, 181–86
Micronutrient requirements, 43–44, 161–72
Miller, C. W., 79
Mineral additives, 164–67
Mochizuki, J., 124, 127
Moderate-nitrogen standard formulas, 129, 132–33

Modular diets, 175
Moore, Ernest E., 78–101
Moore, Frederick A., 78–101
Moss, G., 79
Mucosal barrier, failure of, 8, 15, 16–17, 19, 29, 31–33
Mullen, J. L., 143
Multiple organ system failure syndrome (MOFS), 26, 27, 29–32, 50, 85–86
Multivitamin additives, 168–71

N

Nasojejunal tubes, 66
Needle catheter jejunostomy, 65–66, 92–96
Neurovascular factors in epithelial cell growth, 4
New England Deaconess Hospital (NEDH), 64
Nirgiotis, Jason G., 15–21
Nucleotides, 51–52
Nutritional assessment, 38–39
Nutritional requirements, 37–44
  caloric, 39–40, 156–58
  macronutrients, 40–43, 157–59
  micronutrients, 43–44, 161–72
  modality criteria, 38
  nutritional assessment and, 38–39
  pharmacologic nutrients, *see* Pharmaconutrition

O

Opium, deodorized tincture of, 189, 190
Oral intake
  transition from parenteral nutrition to, 109–10
  transition from tube feeding to, 111–13, 200, 203
Oxygen delivery, 5–6
Oxygen extraction, 5, 6

P

Page, C. P., 79, 86
Palacio, J. C., 129
Palade, G. E., 6

Pancreaticobiliary secretions, 4
Papain, 197–98
Paralytic ileus, 26
Parenteral nutrition, 37, 63–65, 69–70, 80, 87–91, 94–98
  transition to enteral tube feedings, 108–9, 204
  transition to oral intake, 109–10
Park, Roswell, 79
Pasulka, Patrick S., 115–36
Patient selection criteria, 64–65, 155–56
Percutaneous tube placement, 196
Peters, A. L., 124
Pharmaconutrition, 47–54
  arginine, 19–20, 48–49
  glutamine, 19, 28, 32, 49–51
  nucleotides, 51–52
  structured lipids, 52–54
Phosphorus additives, 166–67
Polymeric formulas, 65, 174, 202
Polymorphonuclear leukocytes (PMN), 7–9
Polyunsaturated fatty acids, 52
Postoperative feeding, early, 78–101
  case study, 98–100
  future considerations, 100–101
  historical perspective, 78–80
  injury stress response, 80–81
  metabolic assessment and risk stratification, 82–85
  protocol for, 91–98
  rationale for early nutritional support, 85–91
  substrate demands, 81–82
Potassium additives, 161, 171–72
Prealbumin, 82–83, 89, 90
Predigested (elemental) formulas, 65, 116, 118, 135, 136, 174, 202
Prostanoids, 53
Protein-calorie malnutrition, 18–19
Protein formulas, 127, 129, 130, 132
Protein requirements, 40–42, 157–59
Pulmocare, 122, 124, 125
Pulmonary formulas, 122, 124
Purines, 51
Pyrimidines, 51

Q

Queen, Patricia M., 107–13

R

Rawsen, A. J., 79
Reabilan, 116, 118
Rees, R. G. P., 108
Refeeding syndrome, 181–86
Renal formulas, 120, 121, 123
Respiratory quotient, 122, 124
Retinol-binding protein, 82–83
Reynolds, J. V., 49
Rhode, C. M., 80
Rombeau, John L., 25–34, 129
Rose, W. C., 80
Rush, B., 16–17

S

Saito, H., 20, 49
Scheppach, W., 129
Secretory IgA, 19
Seidner, Douglas L., 3–11
Selective gut decontamination, 20
Sepsis, 9–10, 15–21, 27, 29, 31–33
Sepsis formulas, 127, 128
Serog, P., 122
Serum albumin, 82
Shanbhogue, L. K. R., 40
Shikora, Scott A., 37–44
Short-chain fatty acids (SCFA), 28
Silk, D. B. A., 129
Sodium additives, 161, 171
Souba, W. W., 50
Steele, Kirth W., 3–11
Stools, blood in, 131
Stress gastritis, 30
Structured lipids, 52–54
Surgical tube placement, 193, 194
Swails, Wendy, 69–76, 142–50, 161–72
Systemic response to gut injury, 8–10

T

Teo, T., 54
Thibault, Ann, 197–98
Thomas, Shanthi, 188–92
Thromboxanes, 53
Total enteral nutrition (TEN), 87–91, 94

Total parenteral nutrition (TPN), 37, 63–65, 69–70, 80, 87–91, 94–98
Transitional feeding, 107–13, 199–205
  modalities of, 201
  one tube feedilng formula to another, 110, 199, 201–2
  parenteral to enteral, 108–9
  parenteral to oral intake, 109–10
  preparing patient for discharge, 203, 205
  tube feeding to oral diet, 111–13, 200, 203
Translocation
  defined, 8
  See also Bacterial translocation
Transnasal tube placement, 193, 195
Trauma formulas, 127, 128
Travasorb-Hepatic, 119, 121
Triglyceride digestion, 3–4
Trujillo, Elaine B., 107–13, 199–205
Tube feeding orders, sample, 175, 179–80
Tube feedings
  preparing patient for discharge, 203, 205
  transition between, 110, 199, 201–2
  transition from parenteral to enteral, 108–9
  transition to oral diet, 111–13, 200, 203
  See also Enteral feeding technique
Tumor necrosis factor (TNF), 9–10, 81

V

Valine, 41–42
Van Buren, C. T., 50–52
Vancomycin, 189
Vascular disease, 64
Vital, 42, 176
Vitamin additives, 162–164
Vivonex, 42, 116, 124, 176

W

Weiner, M., 52
Wilmore, Douglas J., 81
Winkler, M. F., 109
Wolfe, R. R., 42
Wren, Christopher, 79

X

Xanthine oxidase-derived oxidants, 17

Z

Ziegler, T. R., 17
Zinc additives, 167
Zonula occludens, 6–7